EDUCATING HEALTH PROFESSIONALS TO ADDRESS THE SOCIAL DETERMINANTS OF MENTAL HEALTH

PROCEEDINGS OF A WORKSHOP

Patricia A. Cuff and Erin Hammers Forstag, *Rapporteurs*

Global Forum on Innovation in Health Professional Education

Board on Global Health

Health and Medicine Division

The National Academies of
SCIENCES · ENGINEERING · MEDICINE

THE NATIONAL ACADEMIES PRESS
Washington, DC
www.nap.edu

THE NATIONAL ACADEMIES PRESS 500 Fifth Street, NW Washington, DC 20001

This activity was supported by contracts between the National Academy of Sciences and Academic Collaborative for Integrative Health, Academy of Nutrition and Dietetics, Accreditation Council for Graduate Medical Education, Aetna Foundation, American Academy of Nursing, American Association of Colleges of Osteopathic Medicine, American Board of Family Medicine, American College of Obstetricians and Gynecologists, American Council of Academic Physical Therapy, American Dental Education Association, American Medical Association, American Nurses Credentialing Center, American Occupational Therapy Association, American Osteopathic Association, American Physical Therapy Association, American Psychological Association, American Speech-Language-Hearing Association, Association of American Medical Colleges, Association of American Veterinary Medical Colleges, Association of Schools and Colleges of Optometry, Association of Schools of Advancing Health Professions, Athletic Training Strategic Alliance, Council on Social Work Education, The George Washington University, Heron Therapeutics, Josiah Macy Jr. Foundation, Michigan Center for Interprofessional Education, National Academies of Practice, National Association of Social Workers, National Board for Certified Counselors, Inc. and Affiliates, National Board of Medical Examiners, National Council of State Boards of Nursing Inc., National League for Nursing, Physician Assistant Education Association, Society for Simulation in Healthcare, University of Toronto, U.S. Department of Veterans Affairs, and Weill Cornell Medicine–Qatar. Any opinions, findings, conclusions, or recommendations expressed in this publication do not necessarily reflect the views of any organization or agency that provided support for the project.

International Standard Book Number-13: 978-0-309-67293-1
International Standard Book Number-10: 0-309-67293-7
Digital Object Identifier: https://doi.org/10.17226/25711

Additional copies of this publication are available from the National Academies Press, 500 Fifth Street, NW, Keck 360, Washington, DC 20001; (800) 624-6242 or (202) 334-3313; http://www.nap.edu.

Printed in the United States of America

Suggested citation: National Academies of Sciences, Engineering, and Medicine. 2020. *Educating health professionals to address the social determinants of mental health: Proceedings of a workshop*. Washington, DC: The National Academies Press. https://doi.org/10.17226/25711.

The National Academies of
SCIENCES · ENGINEERING · MEDICINE

Consensus Study Reports published by the National Academies of Sciences, Engineering, and Medicine document the evidence-based consensus on the study's statement of task by an authoring committee of experts. Reports typically include findings, conclusions, and recommendations based on information gathered by the committee and the committee's deliberations. Each report has been subjected to a rigorous and independent peer-review process and it represents the position of the National Academies on the statement of task.

Proceedings published by the National Academies of Sciences, Engineering, and Medicine chronicle the presentations and discussions at a workshop, symposium, or other event convened by the National Academies. The statements and opinions contained in proceedings are those of the participants and are not endorsed by other participants, the planning committee, or the National Academies.

For information about other products and activities of the National Academies, please visit www.nationalacademies.org/about/whatwedo.

PLANNING COMMITTEE ON STRENGTHENING THE CONNECTION BETWEEN HEALTH PROFESSIONS EDUCATION AND PRACTICE[1]

KENNITA R. CARTER (*Co-Chair*), Health Resources and Services Administration
CARL SHEPERIS (*Co-Chair*), Texas A&M University–San Antonio
COL. DAVID BENEDEK, Uniformed Services University of the Health Sciences
JULIAN FISHER, Hannover Medical School
MILDRED JOYNER, National Association of Social Workers
ROBERT KEEFE, University at Buffalo School of Social Work
KATHLEEN KLINK, Veterans Health Administration
WENDI SCHWEIGER, National Board for Certified Counselors
ZOHRAY TALIB, California University of Science and Medicine
STEPHANIE TOWNSELL, American Osteopathic Association

Consultants

SANDRA CREWE, Howard University
SANDRA D. LANE, Syracuse University
KENYA MCRAE, American Osteopathic Association
ANGELO MCCLAIN, National Association of Social Workers
ROBERT URSANO,* Institute for Healthcare Improvement

*Assisted in planning but unable to attend the workshop.

---

[1] The National Academies of Sciences, Engineering, and Medicine's planning committees are solely responsible for organizing the workshop, identifying topics, and choosing speakers. The responsibility for the published Proceedings of a Workshop rests with the workshop rapporteurs and the institution.

Reviewers

This Proceedings of a Workshop was reviewed in draft form by individuals chosen for their diverse perspectives and technical expertise. The purpose of this independent review is to provide candid and critical comments that will assist the National Academies of Sciences, Engineering, and Medicine in making each published proceedings as sound as possible and to ensure that it meets the institutional standards for quality, objectivity, evidence, and responsiveness to the charge. The review comments and draft manuscript remain confidential to protect the integrity of the process.

We thank the following individuals for their review of this proceedings:

DARRIN D'AGOSTINO, Kansas City University of Medicine and Biosciences
EMILIA IWU, Rutgers University
SANDRA D. LANE, Syracuse University

Although the reviewers listed above provided many constructive comments and suggestions, they were not asked to endorse the content of the proceedings, nor did they see the final draft before its release. The review of this proceedings was overseen by DANIEL MASYS, University of Washington. He was responsible for making certain that an independent examination of this proceedings was carried out in accordance with standards of the National Academies and that all review comments were carefully considered. Responsibility for the final content rests entirely with the rapporteurs and the National Academies.

Contents

1

Introduction[1]

Highlights

- It is not just the physical health or the mental health of a person that requires support; moving forward, health professionals must bring together the mind and body so learners and practitioners can recognize the importance of caring for the whole person. (Sheperis)
- There is limited training on mental health incorporation in health professional education outside of the training of mental and behavioral health professionals. (Sheperis, Talib)

This list is the rapporteurs' summary of the main points made by individual speakers (noted in parentheses), and the statements have not been endorsed or verified by the National Academies of Sciences, Engineering, and Medicine. They are not intended to reflect a consensus among workshop participants.

---

[1] The planning committee's role was limited to planning the workshop, and the Proceedings of a Workshop was prepared by the rapporteurs as a factual account of what occurred at the workshop. Statements, recommendations, and opinions expressed are those of individual presenters and participants and are not necessarily endorsed or verified by the National Academies of Sciences, Engineering, and Medicine. They should not be construed as reflecting any group consensus.

The social determinants of mental health (SDMH), as recognized by the World Health Organization and the Calouste Gulbenkian Foundation, involve the economic, social, and political conditions into which one is born that influence a person's mental health—and, in particular, that affect the likelihood a person raised in deficient or dangerous conditions often associated with poverty will develop persistent mental health challenges throughout his or her life (WHO and Calouste Gulbenkian Foundation, 2014). This definition was part of a background paper presented on January 11, 2019, by Zohray Talib of the California University of Science and Medicine and Carl Sheperis, formerly with the National Board for Certified Counselors, at the information-gathering session held in Irvine, California, in preparation for a workshop of the Global Forum on Innovation in Health Professional Education. The information gathering was intended to provide members of the workshop planning committee with an opportunity to gain a better understanding of stakeholder views on educating health professionals to address the SDMH. Conversations that took place during the sessions were framed by the Statement of Task (see Box 1-1), which would form the foundation of the workshop on this topic taking place in Washington, DC, on November 14–15, 2019.

In setting the stage for the information gathering, Sheperis pointed out that not all individuals raised in poverty would necessarily experience the mental trauma often associated with being affected by the social determinants of health; however, he did acknowledge the work of Patel and Kleinman, who, as set forth in the background paper, linked mental disorders with low levels of education and inadequate housing, both of which are likely results of poverty (Patel and Kleinman, 2003). Talib expanded the conversation by introducing health professional education. A growing awareness of the negative impacts of the social determinants of health, she remarked, has led many health professional educators to incorporate the social determinants of health into their learning activities.

BOX 1-1
Statement of Task

A planning committee will plan and conduct a 1.5-day public workshop to explore how health professions education and practice organizations and programs are currently addressing social determinants that contribute to mental health disparities across the lifespan. The workshop will also set the stage for discussions on how disparities can affect the mental health and well-being of patients, families, communities, and care providers across the learning continuum.

Sheperis and Talib both emphasized the lack of mental health incorporation into health professional education, outside of the mental and behavioral health professions. Participants at the information-gathering session offered their perspectives on the SDMH, which ranged from psychological trauma experienced by individuals living in underserved communities to mental health challenges faced by practitioners, educators, and learners that often go un- or under-addressed.

Sheperis concluded the information-gathering session by reflecting on what he heard. It is not just the physical health or the mental health of a person that requires support, he said; moving forward, we must bring the mind and the body together so that learners and all practitioners recognize the importance of caring for the whole person. Making sure that health professional educators call out the mental health challenges in their education on the social determinants of health is one potential way to better ensure that mental health is not neglected (see Box 1-2 for an example of a community–education partnership). The current and next generation of providers, Sheperis said, must be made aware of the potential physical and mental health challenges faced by all persons affected by the social determinants of health, as well as of their own mental health vulnerabilities. This orientation formed the basis for the planning of this workshop, which was titled Educating Health Professionals to Address the Social Determinants of Mental Health.

WORKSHOP OBJECTIVES

Carl Sheperis, dean of the College of Education and Human Development at Texas A&M University–San Antonio, opened the workshop by introducing the participants to the overall objective of the workshop: "to understand the mental and physical health impacts of being exposed to the social determinants from macro and meso levels so the knowledge can be applied in a micro level." For this workshop, he said, the *macro* involves work and education aimed at influencing higher-level policy decisions. The other two levels directly target education, with the *meso* focusing on how to provide effective education on the SDMH and the *micro* being the content of that education.

Each of the three levels would purposefully address mental health. Sheperis explained that the workshop was placing particular emphasis on the mental health aspects of the social determinants of health for two reasons. First, compared with physical health, mental health generally does not receive adequate attention, particularly as it relates to social determinants. Second, mental and physical health are inextricably linked and are negatively affected by the violence and trauma that can stem from the dangerous or substandard living conditions frequently associated with

BOX 1-2
Bringing Students into the Community

Timothy "Noble" Jennings-Bey, Chief Executive Officer
Street Addiction Institute Inc., Syracuse, NY

Street Addiction Institute Inc. has educated more than 1,000 Syracuse University students by bringing them out of the classroom and into the community to hear from people like Timothy "Noble" Jennings-Bey, the chief executive officer of Street Addiction Institute Inc. and Mothers Against Gun Violence, a grassroots activist group addressing violence in at-risk neighborhoods. According to Nobel, his hometown of Syracuse in upstate New York is one of the most at-risk cities in the United States. Street Addiction Institute Inc. was set up in 2015 to focus on community violence and trauma in Syracuse. Noble, who is director of the trauma response team for the City of Syracuse, said his team responds to shootings and homicides on a 24-hour basis. "This is not a job for me," he said. "It's a ministry."

These are messages that Noble shares with students to underscore his theory that the streets have an addictive nature, just like cocaine, alcohol, or gambling. Individuals reared in that process are in need of respite and rehabilitation before Noble and others like him can mainstream them back into any educational process or career path. Noble said he understands all too well the lure of "street addiction," having grown up in "one of the worst zip codes in the city of Syracuse." He describes existing between two parallel universes. One is the world of academia, while the other echoes the voices of his peers, many of whom have been murdered in the prison system. In his role as an educator, Noble said, he offers messages that range from getting students to understand what it is like growing up in these traumatized zip codes to inspiring young people from his zip code to aim for goals in the world of academia that they might not ever have thought were possible.

Noble said he disagrees with those who argue that "because you're from a different culture or community, there's no way you can understand what I'm going through." Regardless of where you are coming from, he said, "we all have stories to tell," and some of these stories are rooted in trauma. You do not know what people have been through to get here in this time and in this space, he said, "so a simple gesture of 'Good morning,' and I just humanized this entire space and gave credence to my existence." That is one of the ways and one of the strategies that Noble said he uses to take some of the burden off of young people. While a warm greeting sets the tone, it is the honest sharing of experiences—past and present—among communities, educators, and learners that builds relationships and starts the healing process, because, in the words of Noble, "we all need each other to heal."

SOURCE: Presented by Timothy "Noble" Jennings-Bey on November 14, 2019.

poverty. The economic conditions, as well as the social and political circumstances in which a person is born, are what form the social determinants of health and the mental health challenges that people face throughout their lives. For the purposes of this workshop, Sheperis said, the term "mental health" includes a range of conditions from basic human functioning and wellness to severe mental health disorders.

Following these foundational remarks, Sheperis then introduced the participants to the learning objectives of the workshop (see Box 1-3). He stressed that the workshop was designed for active participation, and he encouraged the audience to think critically about what they would like to learn at the workshop, what personal experiences they brought to the workshop, and how they would move forward to integrate the social determinants of mental health into health professional education. Kennita Carter, medical officer at the Health Resources and Services Administration who worked with Sheperis in establishing the framing of the workshop, added that the planning committee hoped the workshop participants would collectively contribute to the development of a "train the trainer" educational module to address the social determinants of mental health from social, political, and economic perspectives. Carter then shared a story about how she first realized that one person—in her case a teenager growing up

---

BOX 1-3
Learning Objectives of the Workshop

After this workshop, participants will be able to do the following:

1. Understand the impact of the social determinants of mental health across the lifespan
2. Understand how mental health can be incorporated into the health professional education framework for the social determinants of health
3. Differentiate the impact of the social determinants on physical and mental health at macro, meso, and micro levels
4. Examine opportunities to expand health professional education to incorporate the social determinants of mental health
5. Identify experiential learning opportunities related to the social determinants of mental health for health professional education
6. Design a framework for delivering education on the social determinants of mental health to health professionals in training
7. Implement strategies for health professional education that incorporate the social determinants of mental health

SOURCE: Presented by Carl Sheperis on November 15, 2019.

in Los Angeles—can affect social and political discourse, in this case by rallying friends, making posters, and marching to city hall in protest of injustices. Her reason for sharing the story, she said, was to get participants to think about how they, or people they know, may have similarly brought attention to an important issue and to consider how they might apply lessons learned from such experiences to the education of health professionals on the SDMH.

The 1.5-day workshop included presentations on a series of topics as well as small group and breakout group discussions. These small group discussions allowed participants to engage with colleagues from other professions and across sectors, while encouraging in-depth exploration of the topics. Appendix B lays out the agenda set up by the workshop planning committee (see page v for the list of planning committee members). This Proceedings of a Workshop follows the general structure of the agenda. Chapter 2 summarizes the presentations and conversations on understanding the SDMH across the lifespan. It also includes a discussion on effective educational methods on the SDMH for faculty and other health professional educators. Chapter 3 explores how to build and recruit a health workforce to address the SDMH. Chapter 4 captures the presentations and conversations about how to create and improve community-engaged experiential learning opportunities. Chapter 5 summarizes discussions on the importance and impacts of mental health policy and includes a section on interprofessional policy and advocacy training among students. This final chapter ends with messages expressed by individual participants underlining the need for faculty to provide learners with interprofessional policy and advocacy training. Any suggestions made throughout the workshop and captured in this proceedings were made by individual participants and should not be interpreted as consensus opinions or recommendations.

REFERENCES

Patel, V., and A. Kleinman. 2003. Poverty and common mental disorders in developing countries. *Bulletin of the World Health Organization* 81(8):609–615. https://www.ncbi. nlm.nih.gov/pmc/articles/PMC2572527/pdf/14576893.pdf (accessed January 22, 2020).
WHO (World Health Organization) and Calouste Gulbenkian Foundation. 2014. *Social determinants of mental health*. World Health Organization. https://apps.who.int/iris/bitstream/ handle/10665/112828/9789241506809_eng.pdf;jsessionid=0038B0C30674BF3E2FB51 AA66F11B74F?sequence=1 (accessed January 28, 2020).

2

The Social Determinants of Mental Health

Highlights

- The social determinants of mental health (SDMH) deserve equal attention to the social determinants of physical health because mental health conditions have high costs, prevalence, morbidity, and mortality, and they have been neglected in conversations about social determinants. (Shim)
- All policies have an impact on people's mental and physical health, and health professionals have a responsibility to advocate for policies that will improve health. (Shim)
- Contained in the National Academies report *A Framework for Educating Health Professionals to Address the Social Determinants of Health* was the need to emphasize experiential learning that is interprofessional and cross-sectoral. (Fisher)
- Both learners and practitioners need to practice in such a way that acknowledges and addresses the SDMH, or the health professions will never get beyond where they are now. (Klink)
- One of the challenges [to using a team-based model of care] was trying to change the dynamics of a team of health professionals who are used to working parallel to each other in silos. Policy issues will have to be addressed if a sustainable interprofessional environment that bridges academia and practice is to be created. (Carter)

- As educators seek to bring the SDMH into the classroom, it is important that they examine their own biases, conscious and unconscious, in order to better guide their students toward addressing disparities that can increase joy in their patients' lives. (Crewe)

This list is the rapporteurs' summary of the main points made by individual speakers (noted in parentheses), and the statements have not been endorsed or verified by the National Academies of Sciences, Engineering, and Medicine. They are not intended to reflect a consensus among workshop participants.

SOCIAL DETERMINANTS

Following the brief opening remarks, Kennita Carter, senior advisor in the Division of Medicine and Dentistry at the Health Resources and Services Administration, then welcomed the first speaker, Ruth Shim, professor in cultural psychiatry at the University of California (UC), Davis, who co-authored a publication titled *Addressing the Social Determinants of Mental Health: If Not Now, When? If Not Us, Who?* (Shim and Compton, 2018).

During her residency training, Shim said, she noticed something interesting about her patients. She rotated between Emory University Hospital, where many patients are financially well off, and Grady Hospital in downtown Atlanta, where there is a high percentage of homeless and low-income patients. Patients were admitted with the same mental health issues, and they received the same care and services. However, patients from Emory University Hospital tended to get better, while patients from Grady Hospital did not, and Shim "could not figure out what was happening." This experience, Shim said, took her on a journey to understand this disparity and eventually led her to the social determinants of mental health (SDMH).

Before delving deeply into the SDMH, Shim wanted the workshop participants to understand the basic tenets of the social determinants of health (SDH). She defined the SDH as "those factors that impact upon health and well-being: the circumstances into which we are born, grow up, live, work, and age, including the health system" (CSDH, 2008). She added that these factors are shaped by the distribution of money, power, and resources and that the distribution of these resources is influenced by policy choices that are made at global, national, and local levels.

The SDH, Shim said, are predominantly responsible for the health disparities and health inequities that are seen both within and between countries. These terms—"disparities" and "inequities"—are often confused, although they are distinct concepts:

Health disparities: Differences in health status among distinct segments of the population, including differences that occur by gender, race or ethnicity, education or income, disability, or living in various geographic localities.

Health inequities: Disparities in health that are a result of systemic, avoidable, and unjust social and economic policies and practices that create barriers to opportunity.

Health disparities, Shim said, are not associated with a value judgment; they are merely differences in health outcomes between groups. Health inequities, on the other hand, are unjust, avoidable, and due to systemic issues and policy choices. Shim illustrated health inequities with an example from Health Canada illustrating how a toddler's "Why?" questioning can illustrate the social determinants of health (see Box 2-1). This story, said Shim, shows how the boy's hospital visit has far more to do with social and

---

BOX 2-1
Social Determinants and Health Outcomes

Why is Jason in the hospital?
  Because he has a bad infection in his leg.

But why does he have an infection?
  He has a cut on his leg and it got infected.

But why does he have a cut on his leg?
  He was playing in a junk yard next to his apartment building and fell on some sharp, jagged steel there.

But why was he playing in a junk yard?
  His neighborhood is run down. Kids play there, and there is no one to supervise them.

But why does he live in that neighborhood?
  His parents can't afford a nicer place to live.

But why can't his parents afford a nicer place to live?
  His dad is unemployed, and his mom is sick.

But why is his dad unemployed?
  Because he doesn't have much education, and he can't find a job.

But why....?

SOURCES: Presented by Ruth Shim on November 15, 2019; Government of Canada, 2013.

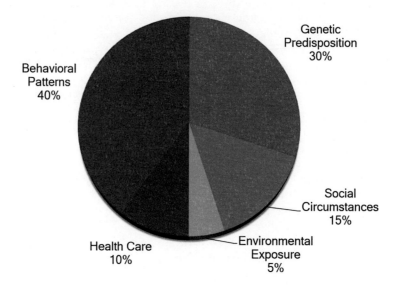

FIGURE 2-1 Determinants of health and their contributions to premature death.
SOURCES: Presented by Ruth Shim on November 14, 2019; created from data in
McGinnis et al., 2002.

economic circumstances—which are related to policies and practices—than
physical or medical issues.

When considering how social determinants influence health, Shim said,
the "ultimate marker of health" is mortality. There are a number of factors
that influence a person's likelihood of premature mortality, including genetic predisposition, behavioral patterns, health care, environmental exposures, and social circumstances (see Figure 2-1). However, Shim said, nearly
all of these factors are ultimately related to social determinants. Exposure
to environmental toxins depends in large part on the neighborhood in
which a person lives and on the availability and affordability of safe housing. Whether a person has access to high-quality health care depends on
income, insurance, and proximity to high-quality facilities. Behavioral patterns—such as exercise, diet, and smoking—are influenced by such factors
as the availability of healthy foods and access to a safe place to exercise.
Even genetic predisposition can be influenced by social determinants; for
example, trauma experienced by parents and grandparents may change the
genetic and epigenetic makeup of their descendants. While some of these
determinants may be due in part to individual choices, Shim said, "the
choices we make are based on the choices we have."[1] People who have
limited options are less likely to be able to make good choices.

---

[1] Quote originally attributed to David Williams, M.D.

The influence of the SDH on mortality, Shim said, can be starkly seen in the different life expectancies of people living in the Washington, DC, metro area (see Figure 2-2). People who live in Montgomery, Fairfax, and Arlington counties—only a few miles away from the city center—have an average life expectancy of 84 to 86 years, while people living in the District of Columbia and in Prince George's County can expect to live to only 78 years, on average (RWJF, 2016). This demonstrates, Shim said, that even small differences in social determinants such as geography can reflect large differences in health outcomes.

Understanding how social determinants lead to health inequities, Shim said, requires attention to the concept of intersectionality. "Intersectionality," a term coined by Kimberle Crenshaw in 1989 to explain the oppression of African American women, refers to the way in which people have multiple overlapping and interacting identities and specifically to the fact that individuals who are members of multiple disadvantaged groups have unique and often compounded disadvantages. For example, a person with mental illness who is also African American and female may face unique challenges that are not addressed by efforts to address the singular issues of mental

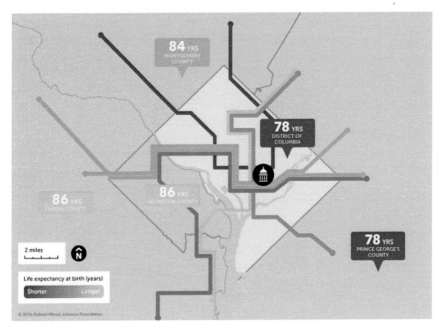

FIGURE 2-2 Life expectancies in the DC metro area.
SOURCES: Presented by Ruth Shim on November 14, 2019. RWJF (2016). Copyright 2016. Robert Wood Johnson Foundation. Used with permission from the Robert Wood Johnson Foundation.

illness, racism, or sexism (Crenshaw, 1989). Shim said that medical students are often taught to "reduce somebody down to one individual, one concept, or one idea," but it is critical to acknowledge the complexities of people and the intersectionality of their various identities.

Mental Health

The SDMH are not distinctly different from the SDH in general, Shim said. However, Shim noted that they deserve special emphasis for three reasons. First, mental illnesses and substance use disorders are highly prevalent and highly disabling. Second, mental health conditions are high-cost, high-morbidity, and high-mortality illnesses. Third, mental health conditions have been largely neglected in conversations and interventions relating to the SDH.

As discussed above, social determinants—such as geography, access to health care, and environmental conditions—are highly influential on health, Shim said, and even seemingly small differences can result in major differences in outcomes. Mental health is influenced by these same social determinants, and the outcomes can be even more severe, she said. People with serious mental illness, Shim said, die on average up to 25 years earlier than the general population. These deaths are not necessarily due to suicide or violence, she said; people with serious mental illness often die of the same causes as everyone else, just earlier. This burden is particularly heavy on people of racial and ethnic minority groups. According to a U.S. Surgeon General's report, these groups have less access to and availability of care, they receive generally poorer-quality mental health services, and they experience a greater disability burden from unmet mental health needs (HHS, 2001). Poor mental health outcomes, Shim said, have been associated with multiple social determinants, including adverse childhood experiences, discrimination, poverty, unemployment, income inequality, food insecurity, and the built environment.

Mental health disorders are particularly difficult to separate from social determinants, Shim said, because conditions are "filtered through the lens of society" and diagnoses are, in large part, based on observations and interpretations of behavior. Behaviors may have different underlying reasons, but these reasons are often not considered when a diagnosis is made. For example, Shim said, a child who is hyperactive and disruptive in class may be diagnosed with attention deficit hyperactivity disorder (ADHD). However, for some children these behaviors may be more readily explained by the fact that the child is hungry. Social determinants such as food insecurity may not only be associated with mental health disorders, but may in fact be confounded with them. Sandra Lane, professor of anthropology and public health at Syracuse University, added a similar observation about diagnoses of behavioral disabilities in children in Syracuse, New York. Syracuse has high rates of violence, and school days are sometimes interrupted by active shooter situations. The schools that have the highest rates of gunshots nearby are also the schools with the highest rates of diagnosed behavioral disabilities, Lane said. However, Lane and her colleagues believe that many of these behavioral disabilities—often diagnosed as ADHD—are actually diagnoses of posttraumatic stress disorder that are due to the violent environment in which the children live and study. Shim concurred and stressed that psychiatric disorders are defined and diagnosed through the lens of experts and their experiences, and these experts may not be familiar with the day-to-day lived experiences of the people who receive these diagnoses.

Social Justice, Public Policy, and Social Norms

Addressing health inequities due to social determinants requires addressing the underlying policies, structures, and resource allocation that create and perpetuate the social determinants. Shim said that mental health inequities are driven by unjust economic policies and practices and that these policies and practices are based on society's collective judgment about "which people are worth advantages and ... which people are worth being disadvantaged." The concept of social justice relates to how resources (i.e., advantages and disadvantages) are distributed in society and attempting to ensure that resources are allocated equally and fairly among all members. Shim provided two ways to think about the concept of social justice. First, David Miller (2003) described it as the distribution of advantages and disadvantages in society and the ways that resources are allocated to people by social institutions. John Rawls (2003) focused on assuring the protection of equal access to liberties, rights, and opportunities and on taking care of the least advantaged members of society.

Shim cautioned, however, that ensuring equal distribution of resources and opportunities is not as straightforward as it may seem. Rather than striving for equality, in which all people receive the same resources or care, we should strive for equity, in which people get the "specific thing that they need to be successful." Shim showed a figure to demonstrate the difference between equality and equity, noting that the people in the illustrations have different needs from one another and therefore require different resources to be successful (see Figure 2-3).

Equity in the distribution of resources and opportunities—and by extension, health equity—cannot be achieved, Shim said, without shifts in social norms and public policy. While politics and medicine may seem distinct, Shim said, they are anything but. As pathologist Rudolph Virchow famously said, "Medicine is a social science, and politics is nothing else but medicine on a large scale." The mechanism by which political choices

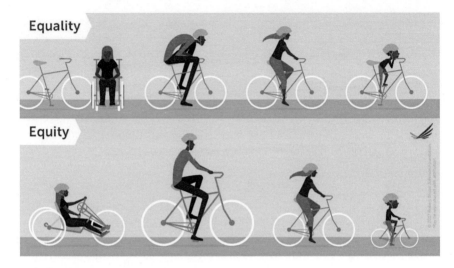

FIGURE 2-3 The difference between equality and equity.
SOURCES: Presented by Ruth Shim on November 14, 2019. RWJF (2017). Copyright 2017. Robert Wood Johnson Foundation. Used with permission from the Robert Wood Johnson Foundation.

affect health outcomes, Shim said, can be seen in Figure 2-4. Social norms and public policy influence one another, and both affect how a society chooses to distribute resources. This distribution of resources affects social determinants such as housing and food security, access to health care, environmental exposures, education, employment, and interaction with the criminal justice system. These determinants, in turn, affect behavioral risk factors, physical and mental stress, and the options that people have at their disposal. These factors then affect mental and physical health outcomes.

Given the intimate relationship between politics and health, Shim said, health professionals have a responsibility to advocate for policies that improve the SDH. "All policies are health policies,"[2] Shim said. All policies have an impact on people's health and mental health, yet "we don't always consider what that impact is before we enact laws." Moving the needle on the SDMH will require health professionals to step outside of their professions and to collaborate across sectors in order to influence and form relationships with elected officials. Shim said that in her profession of psychiatry, many psychiatrists want to stay within the field and only work with other psychiatrists. But to have a true impact, they really need to work with groups outside of the health professions such as police officers,

---

[2] This is a widely used quote that is not original to Shim.

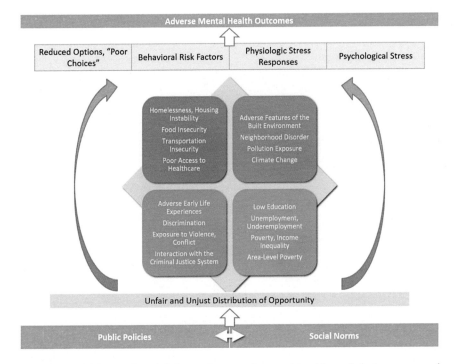

FIGURE 2-4 Types of social determinants of mental health and their causes and consequences.
SOURCES: Presented by Ruth Shim on November 14, 2019; created by Ruth Shim, M.D., M.P.H., and Michael T. Compton, M.D., M.P.H.

teachers, lawyers, and city planners. In addition to working on the local level to affect policy, health professionals need to work on the federal level to increase spending for social care programs. The United States, Shim said, is the only developed country that spends more money on health care than on social care, yet it has poorer health outcomes than other developed countries (APHA, 2020).

In concert with political advocacy, Shim said, there is a need to change the social norms concerning mental health, inclusion, and mutual respect. "We need to create social norms of tolerance, acceptance, and inclusion," she said, and speak up when these norms are not being respected. When people are being "exclusionary, racist, sexist, homophobic, [or] transphobic," she said, "it's on all of us to be the person that speaks up in those situations." Shim closed with a quote from American writer Audre Lorde: "When we speak, we are afraid our words will not be heard or welcomed. But when we are silent, we are still afraid. So it is better to speak."

From Knowledge to Action

In the opening workshop remarks made by Carl Sheperis, dean of the College of Education and Human Development at Texas A&M University–San Antonio, he acknowledged that to guide current and future health professionals concerning their roles in influencing policy-level conversations on the SDMH, health professions educators must first have foundational knowledge concerning the SDH and mental health and on a plan for implementing the educational activity (meso level). To this end, the workshop participants engaged in two sessions targeted at faculty and other health professional educators to explore effective educational methods based on the National Academies consensus study *A Framework for Educating Health Professionals to Address the Social Determinants of Health* (NASEM, 2016).

Julian Fisher, research associate at the Peter L. Reichertz Institute for Medical Informatics at the Hannover Medical School in Germany, presented the framework that was developed by the 2016 consensus study committee and published in that report. The National Academies report also referred to the need to emphasize experiential learning that is interprofessional and cross-sectoral. The next set of workshop speakers addressed this issue. Kathleen Klink, senior advisor in the Office of Academic Affiliations at the Department of Veterans Affairs (VA), and Sandra Crewe, dean of the School of Social Work at Howard University, led participants in a discussion to identify existing and potential opportunities for interprofessional, experiential education on the social determinants of health. More specifically, their focus was on educating the educator on an interprofessional approach to addressing the SDMH through education and action.

FRAMEWORK FOR SOCIAL DETERMINANTS OF MENTAL HEALTH EDUCATION

The SDMH, Fisher said, can be compared to the slope of a hill. Achieving good health outcomes requires pushing a rock up the hill, but the steeper the slope, the harder it is to push (see Figure 2-5). For individuals who have a good income, stable employment, higher education qualifications, secure housing, and good access to food, the slope is shallow, and it is fairly easy to push the rock. For individuals who face greater challenges because of poverty, lack of education and employment opportunities, and lack of access to healthy options, the slope is steep, and it is difficult or nearly impossible to hold the rock steady or push it up the slope. When health professionals ask individuals to make behavioral changes for better health (e.g., eat better food or exercise regularly), people who are already struggling to push the rock will have a much harder time making these

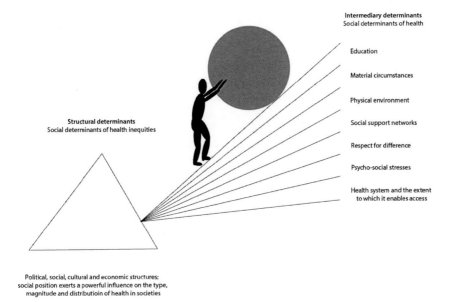

FIGURE 2-5 The impact of social determinants.
NOTE: Intermediary determinants listed (environmental hazards, food/nutrition, housing, employment, education, poverty) based on the World Health Organization Commission on Social Determinants of Mental Health.
SOURCE: Presented by Julian Fisher on November 14, 2019.

changes. In order to truly care for their patients and promote their well-being, health professionals must seek to understand and address the "hills" that their patients are facing. Jody Frost, president of the National Academies of Practice, noted, however, that many of these factors are inter-related and interdependent like cogs in a system and that changing one could have unintended and unforeseen consequences. For example, she said, if a person moves due to poor housing in his neighborhood, the problem of environmental exposures in housing will likely be fixed. However, if as a result of moving the person ends up far from his family, community, and support structures, other problems have been created. Addressing the SDH and health disparities requires a nuanced and holistic view of an individual's social determinants, including how positive and negative social determinants may be intertwined and interdependent, as well as their resources.

Shim's presentation, Fisher said, clearly demonstrated that it is not sufficient to treat people's illnesses without changing the conditions that made them sick in the first place. This suggests an obvious corollary, he added. Like during treatment, it is also not sufficient to educate and train health professionals without having them understand the underlying causes of illness, or the so-called causes of the causes. Unfortunately, educating health professionals to understand and act on the SDMH is not as simple as adding a short module to the curriculum. If, as Shim explained, a large proportion of the contributors to morbidity and mortality are due to social determinants, not to health care, then health professions education must pay an equal amount of attention to the SDH. SDH education, Fisher underscored, must be "mainstreamed" into the curriculum.

Fisher then presented the National Academies' committee's framework (see Figure 2-6). The framework is meant to map out a way to "mainstream" the SDH not just into curricula but also into the lifelong learning journey of a health professional. Zohray Talib, senior associate dean for academic affairs and chair of medical education at the California University of Science and Medicine, added to the conversation, saying that while the framework may be centered around the individual health professional's commitment to lifelong learning, it is also framed by the larger systems-level determinants of education, organization, and community. Incorporating SDH into the health

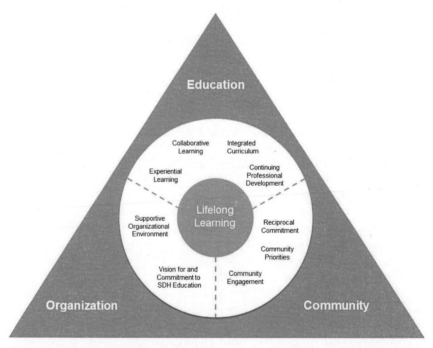

FIGURE 2-6 Framework for lifelong learning for health professionals in understanding and addressing the social determinants of health.
NOTE: SDH = social determinants of health.
SOURCES: Presented by Julian Fisher on November 14, 2019; NASEM, 2016.

professions will require commitment and restructuring of the educational system, collaboration and communication with the local community, and institutional support from organizations to incentivize and support the integration of the SDH into health professions education and practice, she said.

PUTTING EDUCATION INTO ACTION

There is a chicken and an egg issue with education and practice, Klink said. The educational system gives students the skills and knowledge they will bring into practice, but at the same time practice drives what students are learning, particularly in clinical education. Regarding the SDH, Klink said, "without high-quality practice, clinical education is not going to evolve." Both learners and practitioners need to "practice in such a way that [they are] acknowledging and addressing the social determinants of mental health," or the health professions will never get beyond where they are now, she said. Klink gave an example of an interprofessional practice model at the VA that was created in 2010 to address some of the issues discussed at the workshop and which required changes in both practice and education. The Patient Aligned Care Team (PACT) is a team-based model of care in which there are "teamlets" made up of a primary care provider and a nurse as well as an administrative staffer. A broader PACT unit—which includes providers such as pharmacists, social workers, and mental health specialists—provides support to the teamlets. Each teamlet is assigned a group of patients, and the entire PACT team works together to meet the patients' needs, from finding durable medical equipment to setting patients up in community living centers.[3]

In 2011 the VA established the Centers of Excellence in Primary Care Education; five of these centers were selected to teach the PACT model to learners. After a few years of using this model, the VA found that patient outcomes and measures of care were either the same as traditional care or slightly better. In addition, the learners were happy with their experience and felt they were very integrated into their teams. Carter worked in a PACT model and shared her experiences. One of the challenges, she said, was trying to change the dynamics of a team of health professionals who are used to working parallel to each other in silos. For example, it was challenging to convey the idea of dynamic leadership in which each member of the team makes important contributions and the leader of a decision-making process might be any member of the health care team, who could be, but does not need to be, the physician.

Klink and Carter asked workshop participants to share examples of educational models that are or could be useful for preparing learners

---

[3] For more explanation of interprofessional education, see Chapter 5 of the report.

to address the social determinants of mental health, particularly inter-professional models. In response, Fisher described a promising approach used at the Hannover Medical School in Germany called The Patient University. This model uses patients with chronic disease as lifelong learning educators and resource experts on their own diseases and conditions, treatments, and social determinants. This "breaks up the power dynamic" by showing students with and from whom they can learn, and what they can learn from patients through a people-centered learning approach. Each intersection reinforces mutual learning and understanding, with the patients taking new co-created knowledge back out to the community and becoming health educators for others. This unique approach to interprofessional education for collaborative practice, Fisher said, expands the traditional interprofessional team to include the patient and centers the care discussion on the expressed needs of the patient.

Challenges

Workshop participants divided into small groups to further discuss innovative models with an emphasis on the challenges of implementing interprofessional education focused on social determinants. Caswell Evans, associate dean for prevention and public health sciences at the University of Illinois at Chicago College of Dentistry, said that at his university, inter-professional teamwork and education are highly regarded and that leadership and the faculty have a sincere intent to bring this about. However, in actual practice, this commitment is manifested in just 1 day on the undergraduate health sciences campus, where students and faculty get together to discuss case studies in a multidisciplinary way. Evans explained that this day of interprofessional education is repeated annually but has not expanded into any broader efforts to regularly and intentionally bring together learners from different disciplines.

Sheperis reported that many participants at his table felt that many students are participating in a rich world of cross-disciplinary, integrated team training and applied practice opportunities in the academic environment. However, he said, once they move into the professional practice environment, there is a re-segregation of professions. A bridge between the academic and professional experiences is needed in order to continue the integrated team care approach initiated in academia, he said. Similarly, Frank Ascione, professor of clinical and social and administrative sciences at the University of Michigan College of Pharmacy, said that his table discussed the fact that at the University of Michigan Medical School there is a longitudinal, multidisciplinary approach to education that brings together students from 14 different disciplines to share perspectives. However, when students go into the community, the multidisciplinary structure is no longer in place because of organizational, infrastructural, and funding barriers. For example, students are usually mentored or supervised by a practitioner from their own fields, rather than a team approach being used. Carter added some context to these two comments, noting that reimbursement is a major barrier to interprofessional practice. There are disparities in how much different professionals are paid; there are multiple types of reimbursement (e.g., Medicare and Medicaid, commercial insurance, private pay, etc.); there are often separate systems for physical, behavioral, and oral health; and coverage for services and providers varies state to state. These policy issues, Carter said, will have to be addressed if a sustainable interprofessional environment that bridges academia and practice is to be created (see Appendix D for the background paper presented at the planning meeting for bridging the education-to-practice divide in addressing the SDMH).

Potential and Existing Educational Activities

In the second half of the session, Crewe asked workshop participants to take a few minutes to discuss ideas for effective interprofessional educational activities specifically related to the SDH. Afterward, a spokesperson for each set of table discussants reported on the main messages that were discussed by participants in his or her group. General ideas were discussed first, and then specific existing programs were described. Participant Candance Willett said that health educators often use buzzwords like "community involvement" and "community engagement," but "we are really not on the ground like we should be." Doing hands-on work in the community—which means really getting to know the residents and developing a relationship with them—is invaluable to the educational experience, she said. Another spokesperson reported that his group discussed identifying natural opportunities for interdisciplinary learning. For example, instead of students from nursing, physical therapy, and occupational therapy all holding separate anatomy and physiology classes, "why not put them all in the same room?" This model could be effective if dialogue is purposefully encouraged among the health professions and could also be used for community learning opportunities—for example, by having a community member or organizational leader come in and discuss a topic of relevance to the community. As part of these interdisciplinary classes, students could debrief and discuss the material together, thus exposing each other to different perspectives, and perhaps could even discuss how they personally relate to the material. The spokesperson said interactions like these are "where we begin to change the culture."

Refugee Health and Gun Violence

There are two existing programs at Syracuse University in New York that are interdisciplinary and community-based, said Sandra Lane. The first is a course on refugee health, which matches a refugee family with a student from Syracuse University and a health professions student from the State University of New York Upstate Medical University. The students, who come from a variety of health and non-health disciplines, work with the families for a semester and conduct home visits. The second program brings students from Syracuse University into the community to hear about gun violence and its impact on families and the community. Unfortunately, Lane said, there is little support for these programs institutionally. The existence of the programs relies on the perseverance and hard work of community members and faculty members. See Chapter 5 for a further discussion of these programs.

Central Valley Bus Tours

UC Davis, Shim said, runs an activity called the Interprofessional Bus Tour of the Central Valley that was created by Jann Murray-García, M.D., M.P.H. The tour is open to students and leaders from multiple health professions schools, including nursing, medicine, and public health. The tour takes participants into the Central Valley community, where they learn from community members and leaders about the history of the area and how health inequities have developed. One of the fears in such an activity, Shim said, is that it may exacerbate divisions between the students and the community and create a negative perspective about the community. Fortunately, Shim said, many of the students that attend the health professions schools at UC Davis are from the community itself and participate in the bus tours so that they can share their perspective and experiences. In the UC Davis environment, this model of education works primarily due to the commitment of the community leaders and the student advocates dedicated to enhancing the education of peers and colleagues.

Guided Assessments

Reamer Bushardt, professor and senior associate dean in The George Washington University School of Medicine and Health Sciences, shared an example of a powerful interprofessional training experience that he had during a rural family medicine clerkship. The training involved teams of students from different health professions working with patients with mental illnesses and substance use disorders. As learners interviewed and conducted assessments with patients in an outpatient primary care setting, an experienced clinical psychologist was in a control room watching the assessment and could talk to the learner through a device in the learner's ear. This allowed the learner to have an authentic learning experience without "fumbling through" the clinical interaction, because the psychologist would help the learner to understand the nuances of assessment, interpret patient feedback, and probe beyond the clinical into social factors. Bushardt said, "This experience changed my clinical approach to individuals with mental illness, demonstrated the importance of discussing social determinants of health, and instilled a deep appreciation for the expertise of mental health counselors and therapists."

Camden Coalition Hotspotting

Jeffery Stewart, senior vice president for interprofessional and global collaboration at the American Dental Education Association, said that his group discussed the Camden Coalition's hotspotting programs. These programs, which are now all over the country, are designed to help people and communities with both health issues and non-health issues. At the beginning of the development of a program, institutional representatives go out into the community and engage with various organizations and individuals about what the community needs and how the institution could help. Interprofessional teams of learners and other health professionals go into the community, learn from the community, and assist where they can. For example, Stewart said, a dental student might help a community member access housing assistance by getting in touch with the appropriate government agency. The community is put at the center of the program and guides its development and implementation.

Moving Forward

There were several takeaways from this discussion, Crewe said. First, it is essential to invest in team approaches. "This is not a silo activity that we are engaged in," she said. Second, the diversity of the team matters because "new ideas emerge when there are individuals who don't just look like you." Health profession educators need to engage in interprofessional dialogue about the social determinants of health that allows for the voices of many different perspectives and communities. Third, "good things take time." Working on the social determinants of mental health is not a one-time endeavor; it is a process that takes time and effort and requires in-depth engagement among the community, academia, and practice. Finally, Crewe said, social determinants are relevant not only to patients but also to educators and practitioners. As educators seek to bring the SDMH into the classroom, it is important that they examine their own biases, conscious and unconscious, in order to better guide their students toward addressing disparities that can increase joy in their patients' lives.

REFERENCES

APHA (American Public Health Association). 2020. *Investing in the healthiest nation.* https://apha.org/what-is-public-health/generation-public-health/take-action/invest-in-health (accessed January 22, 2020).

Crenshaw, K. 1989. Demarginalizing the intersection of race and sex: A black feminist critique of antidiscrimination doctrine, feminist theory and antiracist politics. *University of Chicago Legal Forum* 1989(1):139–167.

CSDH (Commission on Social Determinants of Health). 2008. *Closing the gap in a generation: Health equity through action on the social determinants of health.* World Health Organization. https://www.who.int/social_determinants/final_report/csdh_finalreport_2008.pdf (accessed January 22, 2020).

Government of Canada. 2013. *What makes Canadians healthy or unhealthy?* https://www.canada.ca/en/public-health/services/health-promotion/population-health/what-determines-health/what-makes-canadians-healthy-unhealthy.html (accessed January 22, 2020).

HHS (Department of Health and Human Services). 2001. *Mental health: Culture, race, and ethnicity—a supplement to mental health: A report of the Surgeon General.* Department of Health and Human Services, Substance Abuse and Mental Health Services Administration, Center for Mental Health Services. https://www.ncbi.nlm.nih.gov/books/NBK44243/?report=reader (accessed January 22, 2020).

McGinnis, J. M., P. Williams-Russo, and J. R. Knickman. 2002. The case for more active policy attention to health promotion. *Health Affairs* 21(2):78–93.

Miller, D. 2003. *Principles of social justice.* Cambridge, MA: Harvard University Press.

NASEM (National Academies of Sciences, Engineering, and Medicine). 2016. *A framework for educating health professionals to address the social determinants of health.* Washington, DC: The National Academies Press.

Rawls, J. 2003. *Justice as fairness: A restatement, 2nd ed.* Cambridge, MA: Belknap Press: An Imprint of Harvard University Press.

RWJF (Robert Wood Johnson Foundation). 2016. *Mapping life expectancy: Washington, D.C.* https://societyhealth.vcu.edu/work/the-projects/mapswashingtondc.html (accessed January 22, 2020).

RWJF. 2017. *Visualizing health equity: One size does not fit all infographic.* https://www.rwjf.org/en/library/infographics/visualizing-health-equity.html (accessed January 22, 2020).

Shim, R. S., and M. T. Compton. 2018. Addressing the social determinants of mental health: If not now, when? If not us, who? *Psychiatric Services* 69(8):844–846.

3

Recruiting and Supporting
a Diverse Workforce

Highlights

- A diverse health workforce, drawn from the community that it serves, is best suited to help the community and patients/clients address the social determinants of mental health. (Horne)
- The Substance Abuse and Mental Health Services Administration states that the Minority Fellowship Program (MFP) was created in 1973 in order to increase the number of ethnic minorities in mental health professions and to provide more culturally competent care to an increasingly ethnically diverse population in the United States. (Schweiger; SAMHSA, 2020)
- The MFP builds on [fellows' shared experiences] by affirming and validating the fellows' life experiences, building a space where fellows can be authentic, promoting self-efficacy, building community, and empowering creativity. (Nguyen)
- The main role of a mentor is forging a path that supports the mentee in achieving as much as possible. (BigFoot)

This list is the rapporteurs' summary of the main points made by individual speakers (noted in parentheses), and the statements have not been endorsed or verified by the National Academies of Sciences, Engineering, and Medicine. They are not intended to reflect a consensus among workshop participants.

In order to effectively understand and address the social determinants of mental health (SDMH), health professionals must be able to understand their patients' cultures, the barriers they face, the opportunities at their disposal, and the context in which they live their lives. If health professionals are drawn from the community that they serve, they will more likely be able to fulfill this role. The Minority Fellowship Program (MFP) at the Substance Abuse and Mental Health Services Administration (SAMHSA) is designed in part to address this issue, said Wendi Schweiger, director of international capacity building at the National Board for Certified Counselors, Inc. and Affiliates. The MFP was originally created in 1973 by the National Institute of Mental Health and later transferred to SAMHSA to "increase the number of ethnic minorities in mental health professions and to provide more culturally competent care to an increasingly ethnically diverse population" (SAMHSA, 2020) in the United States. Organizations representing mental health disciplines apply for grants to support the administration and award of funding for students and new professionals who are committed to providing services, creating policy, and advocating for minority populations.

A total of seven organizations representing the mental health professions administer minority fellowship programs, and three of them were represented at the workshop:

- **The American Psychological Association (APA)** has administrated a minority fellowship program since 1974. The program provides opportunities for guidance through graduate-level and postdoctoral fellowships in areas related to behavioral health services for ethnic minority communities. This program also offers a summer institute and interdisciplinary mentoring for social and behavioral scientists. APA has awarded more than 2,000 fellowship opportunities since the founding of the program.
- **The Council on Social Work Education (CSWE)** also founded its minority fellowship program in 1974, and it has had more than 800 recipients since the program's founding. CSWE's program offers fellowships to doctoral-level and master's-level students who are dedicated to working in practice, research, teaching, and policy on behalf of underrepresented or underserved persons.
- **The National Board for Certified Counselors (NBCC)** is the newest mental health professional organization with a minority fellowship program; it was awarded funding from SAMHSA beginning in 2012. Grants from SAMHSA allow NBCC to distribute both doctoral-level and master's-level fellowships to graduate students, with more than 400 fellowships awarded so far.

These three organizations alone, Schweiger said, have awarded fellow-ships to more than 3,200 mental health professionals with the intention of diversifying the mental health behavior workforce and mentoring professionals who wish to serve in underrepresented populations. In addition to these three, organizations representing nursing, psychiatry, marriage and family therapy, and addiction professionals also administer minority fellow-ship programs.

THE NEED FOR MINORITY MENTAL HEALTH PROFESSIONALS

Workshop participants heard from three individuals associated with the MFP, each of whom discussed the importance of minority mental health professionals. Robert Horne, assistant professor of counselor education and director of the Addiction Studies Certificate Program at North Carolina Central University, said that there are approximately 60 million people with a mental health or substance use disorder, yet there are only approximately 260,000 qualified counselors for this population (BLS, 2019). This equates to about 1 counselor per 230 people with a current disorder. Horne said that this means there are "enough clients for all of us to stay employed" and there is no need for competition among various health professions. In fact, to best serve these clients, professionals should be providing holistic care by working collaboratively with physicians, counselors, psychiatrists, social workers, and others. In addition, only 10.3 percent of all mental health counselors are non–European American, he said. There is a large group of untapped people who could be recruited into the profession, including ethnic and cultural minorities as well as social minorities (e.g., lesbian, gay, bisexual, transgender, queer or questioning populations). People with mental health and substance use disorder are looking for assistance, and "they are looking for people who look like them to serve them." There is a misconception, Horne said, that some minority populations simply do not access some services, such as counseling. Horne said that in his observations as an ordained minister, "it's not so much that African Americans don't go to counseling … they just don't go to you." People tend to go to the cultural institutions that they trust, he said, which is something that should be kept in mind as health professionals are recruited and trained.

Duy Nguyen, director of the minority fellowship program at CSWE, shared his experiences growing up in a Vietnamese immigrant family. Having been raised in a bicultural, bilingual world brought him into the helping professions, he said, and an interaction at summer camp showed him that he had unique capacities to bring to his work. Early in his social work career, Nguyen worked at a summer camp for children with emotional and behavioral disorders, and he met a camper who spoke Vietnamese. Because of their shared language and culture, Nguyen said, she opened up to him in ways that she had not done with other counselors. This relationship convinced him that his upbringing could be an asset and spurred him to pursue working in community mental health with Southeast Asian refugees. He said that this path was not well worn: a professor once told him he would have to make his own way working with this community, and he is one of only a few Vietnamese licensed social workers in the state of Illinois.

Dolores Subia BigFoot is a presidential professor who directs the Native American programs at the Center on Child Abuse and Neglect at the University of Oklahoma Health Sciences Center. She is also an enrolled member of the Caddo Nation of Oklahoma. BigFoot grew up in a rural, poor community and has used her connections and experience to encourage and support young people from similar circumstances to pursue their goals of becoming health professionals and serving their communities.

CRITICAL ELEMENTS

The speakers discussed many elements they identified as critical for recruiting, supporting, retaining, and promoting a diverse workforce, including the following:

- Organizational support
- Opportunity to be authentic
- Support for students and professionals
- Integration with community
- Mentorship
- Community definitions of well-being and success
- Self-care and support

Organizational Support

Building an educational program centered on social determinants and community engagement, Horne said, requires educational institutions to be on board and to be ready for change. Sometimes the institution is simply not ready, he said, but there are ways to move forward anyway. Fellows—such as those from the minority fellowship program—can sometimes "be the change" themselves. Even if an institution is resistant to change and unwilling to offer adequate support, fellows can create networks, connections, and resources in order to sustain a program and keep fellows motivated and supported.

Opportunity to Be Authentic

In his experience as director of the minority fellowship program at CSWE, Nguyen said that he has found that one of the key benefits of the program for fellows is seeing and working with other people like them. While the fellows are drawn from different racial, ethnic, and cultural backgrounds, many of them have shared experiences, and for many, it is the "first time they're in a room with other folks" similar to themselves. The program, Nguyen said, builds on this by affirming and validating the fellows' life experiences, building a space where fellows can be authentic, promoting self-efficacy, building community, and empowering creativity.

Support for Students and Professionals

Recruiting and retaining diverse young people into the health professions requires work on several fronts, Nguyen said. First, there needs to be a clear path to financial stability for students, whether through grants, fellowships, loan forgiveness, or other programs. Second, the economic models of community-based organizations that deal with minority health need to be examined in order to address disparities in grants, contracts, reimbursement, and employee compensation. Minority members of the workforce need to see that there are sustainable and economically viable career options. Third, students need to be engaged early—as early as high school—and to be supported all along the academic pathway. Supporting students includes addressing class and privilege in predominantly white institutions, ensuring that the curriculum is not geared toward educating primarily non-Hispanic white students, and making certain that minority students feel seen, heard, and understood in their institutions and classes. A more diverse faculty—from instructors to deans—can help minority students feel more represented and less isolated, Nguyen said. Finally, Nguyen said that "we cannot assume" that students from minority communities will necessarily "be interested or committed to addressing the behavioral health needs of their community." It will be necessary to recruit and train a larger number of diverse students in order to yield a sufficient number to work in underserved communities.

Horne followed up on this discussion by observing that minority faculty members are few and far between. While more minority students are pursuing doctorate degrees, the number of people of color working in academia "has barely budged," he said. Horne said that he has observed that minority faculty tend to circulate between institutions, starting over every few years when they do not receive tenure. Horne said that when his students or mentees are deciding where to pursue opportunities, he encourages them to look for places where they feel accepted and comfortable and to scrutinize the actual number of minority faculty who are getting tenure because "that's where the rubber meets the road."

Integration with Community

Educating health professionals to address the SDMH, Horne said, requires engagement with and attachment to the local community. A health professions education program must be engaged in volunteering and advocacy in the community, and there must be a relationship of mutual trust so that people can learn from one another and their experiences. Horne cautioned that simply conducting research in communities is not sufficient for true engagement; accurate research requires a "trusting relationship where people will openly and honestly tell you what they think, versus telling you what they think you want to hear."

Instructors can encourage and facilitate this type of engagement by creating assignments that require students to actually get into the field and communicate and network with people in the community, Horne said, adding that there is an "elitist" attitude that community members or clients are simply passive recipients of assistance from health professionals. Given this, he encouraged health educators to promote the idea that both community members and health professionals have things to learn from one another and that they can both gain from the experience of working together. Horne added that community engagement can be accomplished through less traditional means as well—such as volunteering as a coach—and that simply getting involved can help break down the stigma of mental health counseling.

Mentorship

BigFoot discussed the importance of mentoring and said that her life trajectory—from growing up in a poor, rural, multi-generational home to becoming a professor, director, and leader in her field—would not have been possible without mentorship, support, and encouragement from others. BigFoot said that her advisor at the University of Oklahoma, Wayne Rowe, gave her a message that she has carried throughout her career: "We selected you to get into the program, and my job is to make sure that you get out successfully." The main role of a mentor is forging a path that supports the mentee in achieving as much as possible, she said. BigFoot repaid this support by mentoring and encouraging other young people, in both formal and informal ways, she said, and she shared two stories about young women's lives that she has affected. The first was an 11th grade girl from a reservation in Montana who contacted BigFoot 3 years after meeting her on a plane. BigFoot had encouraged the girl to apply for summer classes at Harvard University, and while the girl was not able to attend, she had graduated high school, was working on graduating college and going to graduate school, and was working as an advocate at a domestic violence shelter. The second young woman was 14 when she heard BigFoot speak at a University of Oklahoma Upward Bound summer program. At this event, BigFoot had talked with enthusiasm about her work as a helper and a healer and had described her job as the "most perfect job in the world for me." These statements encouraged the girl, who grew up in rural and poor circumstances that were similar to BigFoot's, to become a child psychologist, and she told BigFoot that her words had sustained her through her high school, bachelor's, and master's degrees and as a Ph.D. candidate.

In her work, BigFoot said, she has had the opportunity to formally mentor and support students and professionals through supervising postdoctoral residents and offering practicum experiences at the Indian Country Child Trauma Center. She has also mentored American Indian faculty, and one faculty member whom she has mentored for about 15 years is now a tenure-track professor with multiple publications and national recognition of her work, BigFoot said. This professor is also a mentee through the National Institute on Drug Abuse's Native-to-Native mentorship program. Part of what BigFoot offers to these mentees, she said, is a cultural lens based on an indigenous worldview, which brings a multi-generational perspective and an understanding of how indigenous people fit into the world and, more specifically, into the professional arena. Nguyen endorsed this idea, saying that while some mentees need specific technical or career support, many are simply looking for an individual who looks like them to show them that there is a path to success and who understands the unique challenges and roadblocks that one experiences as a minority in the field.

Horne said that there is a need to "normalize" the mentor–mentee relationship because this is a society that encourages isolation and independence rather than connection and interdependence. Both mentors and mentees have something to give and something to gain from a relationship, he said, and the profession certainly always gains from people working together and helping each other out. One of the major benefits of having a mentor, Horne said, is that mentors have already forged a path and lit the way for others to follow; young professionals do not have to create the path themselves or travel it alone.

Another important aspect of mentorship, Frost said, is teaching grit, tenacity, and resilience. Frost asked the panelists how they convey these attributes to their mentees and students. Nguyen said that part of it is affirming the mentee's goals and supporting the mentee through the process necessary to meet those goals. In particular, he said, mentors can instill hope by demonstrating their own examples of success and by encouraging mentees to persevere through roadblocks. BigFoot added that people need to learn from a young age how to make decisions for themselves and to understand that there are consequences to the decisions they make. Giving young people opportunities to learn what they are capable of, including allowing them to direct their own actions, can help build grit, determination, and motivation.

Community Definitions of Well-Being and Success

Because exploring the social determinants of health (SDH) and the SDMH requires an understanding of health and well-being, BigFoot discussed the issue of how to define those two terms. While health professionals might have a certain way of thinking about well-being, she said, communities have their own lens through which they think about desirable outcomes. For example, BigFoot said that she asked a room of Native Alaskans how they would define child well-being, and their answer was "smoked salmon." The rituals and traditions of gathering and preparing salmon meant that this community was

> able to come together as families; as family groups, they were able to be together, talk together, work out difficulties, they were able to talk about safety, about food preparation, they were able to tell stories, they were able to go back to a location ... they were able to have times for different kinds of conversations, they were able to move forward and to see the results of their harvest and be able to say we're going to make it through this next season.

Looking through a community lens can help professionals better understand and define well-being for their clients and communities. Mildred Joyner, president-elect of the National Association of Social Workers, added that there is a common misconception that people who have difficult life circumstances cannot be healthy or happy, so it is important to ask people how they themselves would define health or happiness and work from there.

She continued that, in addition to seeking and acknowledging community and patient definitions of well-being, it is important for health professionals to define their own ideas of well-being and what professional success means to them. Horne cautioned that while mentors can help young professionals forge a path ahead, ultimately, professionals are responsible for creating a space for themselves within the profession and for ensuring that the space is in line with their authentic selves. If professionals are authentic and honest with themselves, he said, they will find clients and a practice that give them peace and a sense of purpose. BigFoot added that creating space and being authentic require people to be vulnerable and uncomfortable, but that is where personal and professional growth comes from.

Self-Care and Support

BigFoot talked about her conception of self-care and how to "retain our helpers and healers that we have nurtured" and help them to have balance. BigFoot said that, to her, self-care includes understanding that "each individual is a spirit being with a physical body, capable of emotional reactions, an ability to think and process information, and is connected from self to others by different kinds, intensit[ies], and qualit[ies] of relationships." BigFoot said that the drum beat is a good example of embracing self-care, as it allows for the grounding of the physical body, brings feelings that can wash over prior unpleasant feelings, allows for thinking about sensations, and builds a relationship with the drum and with other people who are invited in by the drum beat.

Darla Spence Coffey, president and chief executive officer of CSWE, thanked BigFoot for introducing the concept of self-care, because health professionals are likely to feel additional stress as they take on the expanded role and responsibility of addressing the SDMH, and they will need to take care of themselves. Coffey urged participants to view addressing the SDH as the responsibility of health systems and of entire teams, not of individual practitioners. Putting the burden on individuals will "be completely overwhelming" and will cause practitioners to retreat, she said. BigFoot added that perhaps the word "self-care" is the wrong word to use because it implies individual responsibility. People in the helping professions need support and resources in order to "do the job at the level they would like to do it."

Launette Woolford, vice president of Northwell Health, added that while focusing on addressing the SDMH of patients and clients is important, health professionals must place equal importance on addressing the mental health of the workforce itself. The workforce has its own social determinants, biases, and mental health issues, and these must also be addressed. Horne agreed and said that there is a stigma in the helping professions attached to seeking help. Health professionals fear being labeled if they acknowledge their own humanity, issues, and concerns, he said. There is a tendency to see patients and clients as "others"—the ones with problems or disorders—rather than seeing everyone as human and susceptible to mental health issues.

REFERENCES

BLS (Bureau of Labor Statistics). 2019. *Occupational outlook handbook*. Bureau of Labor Statistics. https://www.bls.gov/ooh (accessed January 22, 2020).
SAMHSA (Substance Abuse and Mental Health Services Administration). 2020. *About the Minority Fellowship Program*. https://www.samhsa.gov/minority-fellowship-program/about (accessed February 12, 2020).

4

Experiential Learning In and Out of the Classroom

Highlights

- Experiential learning requires a community that is ready and receptive to building partnerships, students who are engaged and motivated to make a difference, and faculty who are committed to doing the hard work to bring communities and students together. (Talib)
- It can be difficult for refugees to open up about their past, so people working with them must take the time to gain trust in order to build a relationship of mutual honesty and openness. (Mouity)
- When building relationships between academia and communities, it is critical that faculty members be intentional and sincere. Communities can sense if an academic is "trying to meet a quota" or check the boxes for community engagement. (Jennings-Bey)
- The students all agreed that community- and project-based classes were preferable to traditional classes but that not all students are passionate about the same things, so schools should offer varying levels of engagement and the ability to choose projects that meet students' interests. (Hamlin, Vencel, Walker)
- An academic could team up with a practitioner in order to run a community-based project giving students the opportunity to learn different aspects of the work from different people. (Shank)

- Community-based learning opportunities need to be flexible, based on community needs and goals, and part of a long-term commitment between communities, institutions, faculty, and students. (Lipman)

This list is the rapporteurs' summary of the main points made by individual speakers (noted in parentheses), and the statements have not been endorsed or verified by the National Academies of Sciences, Engineering, and Medicine. They are not intended to reflect a consensus among workshop participants.

Direct engagement with the community is beneficial for anyone involved in health care, from health professions students to health care executives. As an illustration of the importance of community-based experiences, David Benton, chief executive officer (CEO) of the National Council of State Boards of Nursing, shared a story about working in the East End of London. The people in this community, which is an area of huge ethnic and linguistic diversity, faced a number of challenges when trying to access emergency medical care. The CEO at Benton's health care organization was having a difficult time understanding and addressing these challenges. With the cooperation of community members, Benton took the CEO out into the neighborhood to meet with local people from several different ethnic groups. After his experiences in the community, the CEO said that it was frustrating not being able to understand what people were saying or what was happening. Benton used the CEO's frustration to make a point:

> I said, "Just think about it. You went to visit these communities voluntarily. You are mentally healthy, as well as any of us are, and you found it incredibly stressful and frustrating. Just imagine what it would be like if your wife, your child, was coming into the accident emergency department and you were not able to communicate some of those issues."

Benton said that this experience was life changing for the CEO, and it made him realize the efforts that needed to be made to better serve their diverse communities.

Experiential learning—in which students and faculty engage and interact with community members as teachers—is essential for learning about the social determinants and about a health professional's role in addressing them in practice. Zohray Talib, senior associate dean for academic affairs and chair of medical education at the California University of Science and Medicine, opened the session on bringing education to life in and out of the classroom by describing what experiential learning entails. Experiential learning requires a community that is ready and receptive to building partnerships, students who are engaged and motivated to make a difference, and faculty who are committed to doing the hard work to bring communities and students together. Following Talib's opening remarks, workshop participants heard from speakers representing academia, education, and the community. The speakers talked about how to create and improve community-engaged experiential learning opportunities, each from their unique perspective.

COMMUNITY PERSPECTIVE

Love Mouity moved to Syracuse, New York, as a refugee from Congo-Brazzaville in 2007. He now works as a coordinator for refugee outreach for the Catholic Charities of Onondaga County and also co-teaches an interprofessional class at Syracuse University on refugee health. When Mouity and his brothers first came to the United States, they worked in factories despite coming from an upper class, educated background in their home country. Mouity said that going from a "prestigious life to nothing" was very difficult and that he now seeks to be a role model for other refugees who are going through the same process. The work he does at Catholic Charities helps refugees with multiple issues, including mental health, adjusting to their new surroundings, dealing with culture shock, and becoming self-sufficient. Working with refugees, he said, requires compassion, honesty, and a "mentality of tabula rasa." He explained that it is critical to listen to new refugees and their stories, rather than to assume that their stories are all the same. It can be difficult for refugees to open up about their past, so people working with them must take the time to gain trust in order to build a relationship of mutual honesty and openness. Mouity and his colleagues seek to make sure that the refugees who they help can in turn help others who come after them. Their guiding philosophy, said Mouity, is "ubuntu," which is a South African idea that humans are all interdependent with each other and share a universal bond of humanity.

Timothy "Noble" Jennnings-Bey is CEO of Street Addictions Institute Inc. and director for the trauma response team, which responds to shootings and homicides in Syracuse, New York. Jennings-Bey grew up in Syracuse in a low-income, violent neighborhood, and now serves as a leader in his community and works closely with academics and students at Syracuse University. Jennings-Bey spoke about what it takes to build bridges between the world of academia and the community. He started with a story about a conversation with Sandra Lane, professor of public health and anthropology at Syracuse University. One day, Lane told Jennings-Bey that she did not know a single person who had been murdered. This was foreign to Jennings-Bey, who knows more than 150 people who have been murdered. The only way to connect these two parallel universes, Jennings-Bey said, was in a space of empathy. By working to create an intentional, empathetic relationship, both sides can openly communicate and heal from traumas.

Two-Way Street

Jennings-Bey said that the term "cultural competence" is often used as if it is a one-way street in which students and academics learn about the culture of the community and seek to understand it. However, he said, in his opinion cultural competence is a two-way street in which people on both sides share their cultures and their stories and create a strong relationship. Jennings-Bey said that students sometimes have been told that they cannot possibly understand a community that is so different from their own, but he believes that if people humanize each other, they can understand each other. He stressed that "everybody has their own experiences" and that by sharing these experiences and perspectives, they can build relationships.

Intentionality and Sincerity

When building relationships between academia and communities, it is critical that faculty members be intentional and sincere, Jennings-Bey said. Communities, he said, can sense if an academic is "trying to meet a quota" or check the boxes for community engagement. Rather than being told what to do, community members need the spaces and the opportunity to carry on a dialogue and to solve their own problems. Mouity concurred, saying that "the intention has to be real, not just superficial" and that both sides need to have a willingness to find solutions together. Lane added that academics "have to put the time in" to create relationships that will benefit both the community and the educational institution. She said that while there is a lot of interest in replicating the partnership that has been built between Syracuse University and the community, faculty members do not want to "leave the ivory tower and find parking." It is not enough, Lane said, to simply drop students off at a community organization; faculty members need to make efforts to intentionally get to know community members. In her case, Lane said, these efforts included sharing food with people, inviting people to her home, and attending important family events. Once these relationships have been built, she said, it is a natural next step to work together on issues of community concern.

Jennings-Bey added further context to Lane's remark saying that Sandy's bridge between the community and academia has allowed him to provide a different narrative of the trauma in the community, to publish academic papers on his unique theory about street addiction, and to serve as a role model for young people in the community. He said that his journey allows young people to see a potential path forward, one where they can "articulate the pain of the people" and "help generations that come behind us." Jennings-Bey said that he deals with "miracles" every day, such as when mothers who have lost their children to street violence turn around and help other mothers through the same thing. The relationship that Jennings-Bey has forged with students and academics from Syracuse University allows him to convey and communicate this trauma, grit, resilience, and healing power of his community.

STUDENT PERSPECTIVE

To provide further guidance to educators, three health professions students from local colleges described firsthand experiences they had had in and with communities and offered perspectives on the education they received from those experiences. First, each student offered details about the classes that they had found particularly interesting and useful. Molly Vencel, a junior studying global health at the Georgetown University School of Nursing and Health Studies, spoke about two formative classes she has taken. The first was cultural psychology, which involved students conducting in-depth ethnographic interviews with strangers who were from a different culture than the students. During classroom discussions, the students examined their own cultural biases and looked at appropriate ways to conduct research in the community. Vencel echoed Jennings-Bey's statement that community engagement is a two-way street; she said that the time she spent sitting down with the woman she interviewed involved reflecting on her own cultural experiences as much as her subject's. The second formative course, she said, was global mental health, for which the professor brought in speakers with unique perspectives and duties, ranging from doulas to trauma response teams. Vencel said that learning about mental health from such a broad array of speakers gave her a wider perspective on mental health and the multiple opportunities that exist for prevention and intervention along the lifespan. Her experiences in these classes led her to pursue a summer internship at the Indiana State Department of Health, working in a community outreach program for mothers.

Nigel Walker, who is in the last semester of his master's of health administration and hospital management at George Mason University, told workshop participants that his education on social determinants has focused primarily on the fact that these factors are traditionally outside of hospital or health system control. As a student focusing on hospital management, Walker has learned that even "the best strategy, the best plan, the best facilities" cannot address all of the issues that determine a person's health. For example, Walker said he took a health economics class that taught that people have finite resources and make rational decisions about their use of those resources. This class discussed the fact that if a person lives in a food desert and does not have easy access to transportation, he or she may not choose to spend the time and money necessary to travel to buy healthier foods. Lessons like this, Walker said, emphasize that while hospitals have a role to play in keeping people healthy, the hospital approach alone is "not going to work."

Meghan Hamlin, an accelerated nursing student at the Marymount University School of Health Professions, took a health promotion class that focused on the social determinants of health and health disparities and inequities. The class specifically looked at ways that nurses can affect change by working with and educating patients on actions they could take that could lessen the impact of the determinants of health. This class, Hamlin said, was particularly useful because it helped her apply classroom lessons to real-life practice. Hamlin volunteers for an organization called Remote Area Medical, which provides free medical care to those living in remote geographic locations. This class prepared her, she said, to look at upstream causes and downstream effects, make connections between patients' lives and their health issues, and work with other disciplines at the clinics to help patients.

Hands-on Classes

The students offered their opinions on how to improve health professions education to better incorporate the social determinants of health (SDH) and community engagement. All agreed that community- and project-based classes were preferable to traditional classes that are reading and writing focused. Hamlin said that the hands-on experience makes education "more tangible" and easier to hold onto over the long term. Vencel agreed but said that as a freshman, she likely would have chosen a traditional class out of "fear of the time commitments and the emotional investments" of doing community-based work. She said a good approach may be to give students small tastes of hands-on work in a variety of introductory classes and then allow them to choose more in-depth, community-based work in subsequent classes. Vencel added that not all students are passionate about the same things, so schools should offer varying levels of engagement and the ability to choose projects that meet students' interests.

Real-Life Relationships

The students all emphasized the importance of working with communities and organizations, forming real-life relationships, and having the opportunity to continue these relationships after the project or the class ends. Vencel said that after being highly engaged with community organizations for a semester, she felt like she was "left hanging" after the semester ended, and she would have appreciated "more concrete ways of continuing to engage in the projects." Walker agreed, saying that he would like the opportunity to conduct strategic planning with organizations and to have regular follow-up and continued work with the same organization. For example, he said, rather than just creating a strategic plan and "walking away," students and organizations could build on strategies created in previous semesters or by previous students. Hamlin agreed with the need for more practice in real-life situations, saying that actively applying lessons during school—such as how to build relationships with patients—will help prepare her to apply these skills when entering practice.

Interprofessional Education

Matthew Shank, president emeritus of Marymount University, asked the students if they had had the opportunity to participate in interprofessional education. All three students replied that they had not had much opportunity to learn with or work with people from other professions but that they saw the value in doing so. Walker said that his program has been largely theory and classroom based, so learning with students who participate in more real-life experiences (e.g., working in a clinic) would bring a much needed balance to the program. Hamlin said that a unique aspect of her accelerated nursing program is that everyone comes with degrees from different disciplines and has had different experiences. This allows people with different perspectives to share and learn from one another. However, she said, it would also be beneficial to have collaborative experiences with people who will be working in the health field with nurses. Shank added that another option for interprofessional education would be to have instructors from different disciplines working together with traditional health professions faculty. For example, an academic could team up with a practitioner to run a community-based project, giving students the opportunity to learn different aspects of the work from different people.

Mentoring

A workshop participant asked the students if they had formed any relationships with mentors during their education and, if so, what role the mentor has played in their success. Vencel replied that her professors from the cultural psychology and global mental health courses have both stood out as mentors more than other professors, due in part to the more intensive and involved nature of classes that engage the community. Hamlin agreed and said that her relationship with her clinical instructors has been extremely important in giving her hands-on experience and fostering confidence in her ability as a nurse. Walker said that the new program director at his school has been leading an effort to do more community outreach and that he is excited about the opportunity to get involved in shifting the culture toward this goal.

FACULTY PERSPECTIVE

The reputation of the University of Pennsylvania in Philadelphia has not always been positive, said Terri Lipman, assistant dean for community engagement at the University of Pennsylvania School of Nursing. When Lipman first arrived at Penn, she recalled, she attended a meeting where a community member said, "Penn and Children's Hospital comes into the community, you collect your data, you do your projects, and you leave us with nothing." This message, Lipman said, resonated with her and has guided her community-based work. Lipman displayed a map (University of Pennsylvania School of Nursing, 2019) of Philadelphia that showed the number of community engagement projects across the city (see Figure 4-1). This map, Lipman said, shows not just what they have done, but how far they have to go.

In addition to Lipman's work as dean, she is also a nurse practitioner at the Children's Hospital of Philadelphia working with children with endocrine disorders and diabetes. In her role as a clinician, she said, she has "firsthand knowledge of what happens when we don't address social determinants of health." Children with diabetes from well-resourced families have great outcomes, whereas traditional disease- and hospital-focused interventions have "not moved the needle with underresourced families." A new approach, Lipman said, is sending community health workers into patients' homes; these workers address only the SDH and do not discuss diabetes management at all. Preliminary data suggest that this approach is improving diabetes outcomes, she said. Lipman said that health professionals often think that the answer to poor health outcomes is more education and more intervention from health professionals themselves. However, she said, "professional teams don't necessarily address the issues we need to address," whereas community health workers may be able to move the needle when clinicians cannot. Lipman was also clear that any community-engaged program she is involved with that addresses the SDH also includes mental health. In the community setting, she said, the two cannot be separated.

Exploring Best Practices for Community-Based Programs

Lipman shared the lessons she learned from facilitating and leading community-based programs. First, she said, these types of experiences require flexibility on the part of students, faculty, and institutions. Nursing

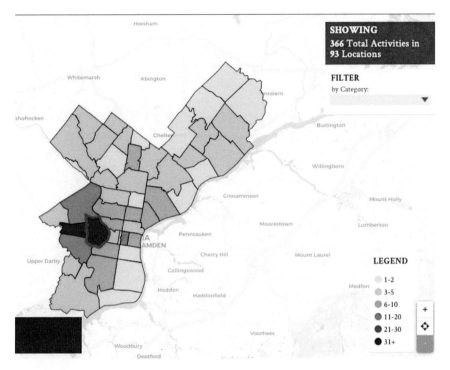

FIGURE 4-1 The University of Pennsylvania School of Nursing community engagement projects across Philadelphia.

SOURCES: Presented by Terri Lipman on November 14, 2019; map licensed by OpenStreetMap, © OpenStreetMap contributors; data available under the Open Database License.

students are accustomed to working in a hospital, where things are quite regimented and scheduled. In contrast, community-based work is less predictable; for example, a high school where a nursing student is supposed to report may be on lockdown due to violence. Faculty and educational institutions must be flexible as well, Lipman said. Community-engaged research and teaching can take an enormous amount of time and effort, particularly when compared with traditional methods, such as giving a PowerPoint lecture. Institutions need to be flexible when making promotion and tenure decisions; community-involved faculty may spend their time and energy on activities that are not traditionally valued but that are key to building strong relationships with the community.

Second, programs need to be community-driven and based on community goals. As an example, Lipman discussed a program she runs called Dance for Health. This program was born out of a community discussion about the community members' desire to have an active, indoor, inter-generational activity that is fun for everyone. The academic and practice partners have a goal of improving health and take health measurements to track progress. The community partners, on the other hand, have said that "what really brings them there is the social support and the relationship building." Still, Lipman said, the community members are excited to track health measurements because they love the idea of improving their health through dancing. The program is co-owned by the community, Lipman said, which means that it continues during academic breaks and is inde-pendent of student or faculty turnover. The program also involves local high school students, who help obtain the health data and then present the data around the country, along with the nursing students. The "heart of the program" is outside of the academic institution, Lipman said, so it is sustainable and community-driven.

The third lesson that Lipman offered is that these programs are relevant for all health professionals, no matter where they end up practicing. Lipman said that she sometimes gets pushback from nursing students who are plan-ning to work in non-community settings, such as intensive care units. These students do not see the relevance of community work to their education. However, Lipman said, the relationship-building skills that students learn in the community are fundamental to providing good health care and to being able to work successfully with patients and families. For this reason, Lipman said, she believes that all students should be exposed to community engagement work, not just those who express an interest in it.

Finally, Lipman said, community-based experiences work best when students and faculty are committed for a long period of time. Rather than doing projects one semester at a time or on a drop-in basis, Lipman's goal is for students to stay with one community experience throughout their education. Lipman said that when entire groups of students come and go, it takes time to rebuild relationships. If students need to leave a project for some reason, there should be a handoff process in order to ensure con-tinuity. Lipman added that faculty also need to be committed; they need to have "the passion and the interest" to engage with the community and to build relationships. If faculty are not fully committed to working with the community, she said, the relationships and projects will not be mutually beneficial or sustainable.

DISCUSSION

Given the enormous benefits and power of experiential learning and community-based work, Talib asked, why are these types of educational opportunities not more readily available? Shank replied that a lot depends on the vision of the university: "If you don't have passion at the top for this, it's not going to work." Even if faculty and students want to do community-based work and are passionate and committed, there are limits to what can be done without buy-in from the university. People at the top of the university or organization, Shank said, need to be consistently talking about community engagement and incentivizing people to carry it out. Incentives could include making community engagement part of tenure decisions or offering community engagement grants. Lane agreed but said that even when leaders are committed to community engagement work, they sometimes do not understand what it takes to actually conduct it. For example, the refugee health class she runs at Syracuse University and at Upstate Medical University involves a great deal of work, including finding families willing to participate, securing funding for stipends for the families, and ensuring that students can get to and from their frequent home visits during the semester. A colleague of Lane's mused about scaling up the program but did not take into account the massive time commitment required for faculty. Newton added that even seemingly straightforward logistical issues—such as housing and bus routes—can derail an experiential learning opportunity if not dealt with ahead of time.

Another reason that experiential opportunities sometimes fail is a lack of intentional and careful planning and management of the project, Newton said. For example, if a student shows up to an organization that is not prepared for that individual, it is a negative experience for both the student and the community, and it can alienate the student from participating in the future. This is a particular hazard when sending students into emerging or worsening crises, such as a community after a hurricane, Newton said. These situations can present opportunities for communities to receive much needed help while at the same time allowing students to gain hands-on experience, but the projects need to be carefully planned and managed so that both sides have a constructive and mutually beneficial experience. An experiential learning project, Newton said, is "not worth doing unless it's done well." Shank added that the expectations of both the community and the students need to be managed, so that both sides understand their roles, responsibilities, and goals. Lipman concurred and noted that students' expectations and intentions are sometimes not aligned with those of the projects; for example, students may want to participate because it will look good on their résumé. Faculty should carefully consider the students who are being sent into experiential learning projects in order to ensure a good match. Lane told a story about this type of issue, in which a student failed to follow through on a research project that the community partner had worked hard on. These types of failures can "burn bridges" in communities, Lane said, and emphasize the need for careful management.

REFERENCE

University of Pennsylvania School of Nursing. 2019. *Community engagement map.* University of Pennsylvania. http://whimsymaps.com/view/sonfacultycommunity_2019 (accessed January 22, 2020).

5

Turning Experience into Policy

Highlights

- Many veterans chose not to use the word "disorder" in the posttraumatic stress acronym, arguing that after what they went through in battle, it would be a disorder not to be affected by the experience. (Moulton)
- In the end, legislation and public policy may help the most—even more than the delivery of quality health care—in reducing inequities that drive mental health outcomes. (Benedek)
- Putting the patient in the center means seeing the whole person—including his or her family, job, community, and unique situation—rather than just his or her medical issue or diagnosis. (Keefe)
- Health professionals need to be prepared and willing to work across sectors if they wish to address social determinants. (Carter)
- Students need to be trained to see "health in all policies" and to advocate for all types of policy on all levels. (Fisher)

This list is the rapporteurs' summary of the main points made by individual speakers (noted in parentheses), and the statements have not been endorsed or verified by the National Academies of Sciences, Engineering, and Medicine. They are not intended to reflect a consensus among workshop participants.

Colonel David Benedek, chairman of the Uniformed Services University of the Health Sciences' Department of Psychiatry, opened the session for the closing keynote given by Representative Seth Moulton, U.S. congressman from the Sixth District of Massachusetts. Benedek remarked that quite a bit of attention had been given during the workshop to identifying the drivers of mental health outcomes stemming from the social determinants of health (SDH). There were also lengthy discussions on the importance of educating health care providers, students, and trainees on these issues and on how they might advocate for changes to improve and reduce disparities and inequities that drive mental health outcomes. It was also stated that, in the end, legislation and public policy may help the most—even more than the delivery of quality health care—in reducing these inequities.

With those few comments, Benedek welcomed Representative Moulton to the stage, asking him to help the forum members and guests better understand how, as educators, "we can teach not only ourselves but our students about our role in trying to work on the legislative process." He encouraged the congressman to share his story and to perhaps remind the audience how, over the course of a lifetime, those drivers of mental health outcomes can change for people, such as how life decisions and circumstances can alter the trajectory of one's mental and physical health outcomes.

Seth Moulton

Congressman, Sixth District of Massachusetts

In response to Benedek's charge and following the path laid by Kennita Carter of the Health Resources and Services Administration in the opening session, Representative Moulton shared his personal journey with mental health stemming from his military service. He also discussed how his combat experiences motivated him to pursue broad-scale changes to federal policy. As background, Moulton said he joined the Marine Corps in 2001 and served four tours of duty in Iraq. After his time in Iraq, he sought treatment for posttraumatic stress,[1] and in 2019 he became the first presidential candidate in American history to openly discuss his own mental health issues. During Moulton's run for the Democratic nomination for president of the United States, he opened up about his mental health struggles, not knowing what the response would be or if it would end his bid for the presidency. The response was "fantastic," he said. Because of his openness, both veterans and non-veterans who had been silent for years told their

---

[1] Moulton said that he, like many veterans, chose not to use the word "disorder," saying that after what they went through in battle, it would be a disorder not to be affected by the experience.

stories and began the process of getting help. Supporting these people in telling their stories, Moulton said, "is the most important thing" that he did while running for president.

Along with sharing his personal story, Moulton developed a three-point mental health plan that he would seek to implement as president. While his bid for the presidency has ended, Moulton said he continues to work on his plan as a member of Congress. The first point of the plan is to establish a national mental health hotline. This proposal has been written into a bipartisan bill that Moulton said has more than 100 co-sponsors in the House and co-leads in the Senate. The second point of the plan would ensure that everyone in the military gets an annual mental health exam, in part because there is a high incidence of mental health issues in the military, but also to emphasize that regular mental health check-ups should be normal and routine for everyone. A related but less comprehensive provision is in the current defense bill; it would ensure that military members coming back from a combat deployment would be seen by a mental health professional within 2 weeks and then would have annual follow-ups. The third point of Moulton's plan is to extend the annual mental health screenings to every high school student in America.

The two main goals of this plan, Moulton said, are to improve access to mental health care and to destigmatize the idea of getting regular mental health exams and seeking additional help when needed. He said that if a person tells co-workers he or she needs to leave early for an annual physical exam, no one bats an eye, but if the same person has to leave early for a mental health appointment, the reaction is not the same. This difference is "fundamentally what we have to change," he said. Moulton added that in the military, seeking mental health care can result in losing security clearance, which means that "some of the people who need care the most are not getting it." If everyone got a mental health exam annually, it would ensure that all military members could get help without fear of being stigmatized or punished. Kimberly Lomis, vice president for undergraduate medical education innovations at the American Medical Association, commented that there are similar issues in health care as well as similar proposals. Health care professionals deal with stressful situations and death on a day-to-day basis, she said, yet seeking help for mental health issues is still stigmatized within the profession. Lomis applauded Moulton's plan and said "the idea of normalizing it and fighting against that stigma is really critical."

In addition to the barrier of stigma, many people—veterans and non-veterans alike—do not know how to access mental health care. Moulton asked the workshop participants if anyone knew the National Suicide Hotline number, and not a single person could accurately recall it. This, Moulton said, is a big problem. "If you wake up tomorrow night and ... your house is burning down, you don't have to go looking for a phone book to figure out who to call," he said. When people are having mental health crises, he continued, it should be just as easy to know whom to call for help. His proposal would make 988 the phone number to call for mental health help and would expand the hotline beyond suicide to all types of mental health issues. Moulton said that many people—including himself—feel as if their issues are not severe enough to warrant reaching out for help. It took him awhile to seek help, he said, because he was not feeling suicidal or having symptoms as bad as some of his fellow veterans. This is a mindset that needs to change, he said, so people can seek help for a range of mental health issues rather than only the most severe.

Implementing some of these proposals, Moulton said, will involve a significant amount of money and require recruiting and training more mental health professionals. While this is a tall challenge, Moulton said, he has learned that "it's better to set the goal and say this is something we want to achieve, and then we'll figure out how to get the people to fill the spots." Pamela Jeffries, professor of nursing and dean of The George Washington University School of Nursing, suggested that school nurses would be excellent partners in the effort to screen high school students. Moulton agreed but said he believes that screenings for both high school students and military members should be conducted by trained mental health professionals, rather than by primary care providers simply asking a few questions during an annual exam.

Some of the solutions that Moulton advocates for on the national level are already being implemented on the state and local levels, said Carl Sheperis of Texas A&M University. For example, he said, Texas has passed a law that requires every classroom teacher in Texas to have mental health training.[2] In San Antonio, one of the poorest school districts in the state, students led a 4-year effort to make a mental health wellness center available for students, parents, and staff (Phillips, 2019). Sheperis asked Moulton how to continue and expand on these types of grassroots efforts. Moulton responded that while there is still a long way to go, the public perception of the issue is changing rapidly. He noted that his mental health provision was passed in the current defense bill with full support from both Democrats and Republicans, which is "incredibly encouraging" for future efforts on both the local and national levels.

Benedek asked Moulton how to get students involved in the political process in order to make changes for mental health on a broad scale. Moulton replied with a story about the first bill that he passed in Congress, which was aimed at using technology to improve access to the Department of Veterans Affairs (VA). A staffer in his office made a video of a fellow staffer, who was a veteran, calling and trying to get an appointment at the

---

[2] Texas Educ. Code § 21.451 and 21.054.

VA but getting caught in an endless loop of automated menu options. The video captured the problem and ended up going viral. Other members of Congress heard about the video—and the issue—from their constituents and reached out to support the bill. Moulton said that members of Congress have a lot of ideas and proposals but that people at the grassroots level, including students, can really influence what gets prioritized (see Box 5-1 for an example of policy priorities impacting mental health).

BOX 5-1
Interstate Highway Policy and Health

As an example of how "all policies are health policies," Congressman Seth Moulton illustrated the link between two seemingly disparate areas: federal interstate highway policy and physical and mental health. The types of communities we live in—literally the physical environment and how communities are constructed—have a massive effect on personal health, he said. New York City has a lower rate of obesity than many areas of the United States, and one of the reasons for this is the fact that people take the subway and walk. "The types of transportation systems that we design influence the types of communities that develop," Moulton said. When people can easily walk or take public transportation, they do so, but when these options are not available, people may have to drive a car to go a few blocks. The difference between these neighborhoods can have a massive impact on individual health. Clearly, people's physical health is affected by how much they walk on a regular basis, but these differences affect mental health as well. For example, Moulton said, if people are out walking in the neighborhood, they are interacting with more people and getting more opportunities to socialize. If a community is built far from other neighborhoods and is only accessible to people of a certain income level, people living in that community will be more likely to primarily interact with people of similar life circumstances. Conversely, a diverse neighborhood brings people of diverse backgrounds together, which can affect people's tolerance and understanding of different perspectives. The priorities that the federal government sets through transportation policy—building roads rather than investing in public transportation—can have dramatic effects on people's physical and mental health, Moulton said, and transportation policy, then, is something that needs more attention.

SOURCE: Presented by Seth Moulton on November 16, 2019.

THE ROLE OF HEALTH EDUCATION IN POLICY

In an attempt to apply previous discussions at the macro and meso levels to specific life situations (micro level), workshop participants gathered in small groups to discuss case studies that were presented by the planning committee as "case histories." These case histories dealt with the role of social determinants of mental health (SDMH) at three stages of life: pregnancy and birth, young adulthood, and older adulthood. Although the planning committee selected these three points in time, Sheperis noted that when using case histories for education, any point along the life course could be used to illustrate how mental and physical health are both affected by social determinants, how social determinants are affected by policies, and how learners can work toward influencing policies. The case histories (see Appendix E) involved patients who presented for care with seemingly straightforward medical issues, but through a gradual unveiling of information it became apparent that each case was affected in some way by the SDH that affected the person's mental health and well-being. Participants worked through the case studies and discussed how the situations could be used in health professions education to encourage thinking about social determinants, how these determinants may influence care decisions, and how health professionals could address the determinants on individual, community, and policy levels.

Participants reconvened to share takeaways from the group discussions as well as from the workshop as a whole. The discussion primarily focused on competencies that educational institutions should seek to instill in health professions students. In addition to the more in-depth conversations summarized next, participants identified a variety of potential areas for educational competencies among faculty members, including the following:

- Looking at how policies connect people with each other and the environment using relational theories
- Assessing community needs and assets that align with community-engaged learning objectives (i.e., bidirectional mutuality)
- Building and maintaining sustainable community projects
- Learning from effective interprofessional, collaborative teams
- Establishing cross-sectoral relationships

Making the Link Between Patients and Policies

Students and health professionals need to learn to put the patient in the center in order to make sound decisions, said Robert Keefe, associate professor at the University at Buffalo School of Social Work. Putting the patient in the center means seeing the whole person—including the patient's family, job, community, and unique situation—rather than just his or her medical issue or diagnosis. Once health professionals see the patient as a whole person, Keefe said, they will be better equipped to care for the patient as well as to potentially address social determinants and mental health challenges through broader scale initiatives. Kennita Carter, senior advisor in the Division of Medicine and Dentistry at the Health Resources and Services Administration, added that health professionals need to be prepared and willing to work across sectors to address social determinants. A patient's needs might be best met, for instance, not through the health sector, but by connecting the patient with housing, food, or other resources or by advocating for change in these areas.

Policy and Advocacy Training

Julian Fisher, research associate at the Peter L. Reichertz Institute for Medical Informatics at the Hannover Medical School in Germany, said that everyone needs a skill set in policy and advocacy training regardless of his or her eventual career path, and that this skill set is "very weak and underdeveloped within the health and social workforce." Fisher said that while there is some attention paid to social determinants on the individual or community levels, there is far less attention paid to the ways in which policy affects structural determinants. These structural determinants (e.g., housing policy) have a major impact on health and well-being and accentuate individual or community determinants. Students need to be trained in "health in all policy"[3] approaches to be able to advocate for health in all sectors and across all levels, Fisher said. In order to do so, he said, students will need skills such as tracking legislation, reaching out to representatives on multiple levels, and advocating for policies in areas in which they are not experts. Carter added that in addition to advocating for new policies, students should be trained to leverage existing policies and resources to make change.

Lomis cautioned that some health professions students will be passionate about advocacy and will pursue it as a major part of their career, while others may be overwhelmed or simply uninterested in the idea of policy and advocacy. She suggested that there be a broad continuum of engagement in advocacy, with a core foundation of advocacy skills in which all students are trained. Mark Merrick of the Athletic Training Strategic Alliance added that simply training students in the mechanisms of advocacy does not create advocates. Students must feel a connection, Merrick said "You create

---

[3] Health in All Policies describes an approach that integrates health considerations across sectors. For more information on Health in All Policies, visit https://www.cdc.gov/policy/hiap/index.html (accessed February 11, 2020).

advocates when you connect students powerfully to issues in which they are invested and want to make a change." Fisher agreed and suggested that one goal of health professions education should be to give all students basic skills in advocacy, so that when students find themselves in a situation wanting or needing to advocate, they can "fire these skills up."

Jody Frost, president of the National Academies of Practice (NAP), stressed the importance of teaching and conducting interprofessional advocacy rather than advocacy based on the needs and structures of a specific health profession. She said that this type of advocacy is "powerful" and that policy makers want to hear about new approaches that are supported by multiple health professions. Kennita Carter, senior advisor in the Division of Medicine and Dentistry at the Health Resources and Services Administration, added that in addition to interprofessional advocacy, students should be taught cross-sectoral advocacy so that they can work together with people outside of the health professions.

Self-Awareness and Self-Care

Part of preparing students to address the mental and physical effects of the social determinants and to advocate for change, one participant said, is helping students learn about themselves and about where they fit in their schools, communities, and professions. When students begin their health professions education, many do not have the skills to navigate the systems they are in and to maintain their physical, mental, emotional, spiritual, and financial well-being. Educators and administrators can help students by giving them the space and the opportunity to process their own life experiences and to reflect on their new experiences as students and health professionals. A second participant suggested that a school could use bereavement and loss as an "entry point" to get students to have these reflections and conversations because many, if not most, students have experienced loss. This led to a third participant commenting that students also need to have conversations about culture, class, race, and ethnicity and about how these intersect and can affect a person's self-care and self-advocacy as well as their care and advocacy for others.

Integrating Social Care

In September 2019 the National Academies released a consensus study report titled *Integrating Social Care into the Delivery of Health Care: Moving Upstream to Improve the Nation's Health*. Darla Spence Coffey, president of the Council on Social Work Education, noted that the report contains a number of conclusions and recommendations that are relevant to educating health professionals to address the social determinants of mental health, including a framework for how interprofessional teams can look beyond clinical interventions toward social needs. The framework included five "As" that are critical to this work. First, the team members must be *aware* of the impact of social determinants. Second, the team must know how to *adjust* care in order to accommodate or address social determinants. Third, the team should offer *assistance* by connecting patients with relevant resources. Fourth, the team should seek to *align* the system of social supports so that professionals are not working in siloes. Finally, team members should have the ability to *advocate* for changes on a broader scale that may affect their patients (NASEM, 2019).

Faculty for the Future and Closing Remarks

Whether a particular faculty member educates students on the role of health professionals in advocating for patients and communities may be influenced by the type of training that educator received himself or herself. This was Sheperis's message as he reflected on a breakout session conversation that he had heard. From the discussion, he said, it appeared that some professions, such as counseling, psychology, and social work, embed advocacy and policy development as part of the training process and that faculty members view it as their ethical responsibility to teach students these concepts and skills. Faculty might take students to a state capitol or to Capitol Hill for advocacy days or train them in how to write letters to influence policy. Students are trained on how to know whom their representatives are and on how to use their "voice" in terms of policy development. In contrast, he said, other health professions with already crowded curricula, such as medicine and nursing, may have examples of such training but, overall, seem to place less of an emphasis on instructing learners on how to do advocacy. Sandra Crewe, dean of the Howard University School of Social Work, was quick to point out that including advocacy training in areas of the SDMH could do a dis-service to the importance of this area by offering inadequate or insufficient training. The challenge for educators is how to offer such training within a crowded educational program. One idea that Crewe suggested was to find ways of integrating advocacy training into already established competency training in order to avoid "spreading ourselves too thinly."

Frost suggested taking an interprofessional approach to advocacy training. In this way, she said, different health professions can learn from each other and can leverage different professions' expertise in offering advocacy training across curricula. Frost underscored the power of interprofessional advocacy as she described her recent experience briefing lawmakers on Capitol Hill who were captivated by NAP's interprofessional approach to addressing challenges in health care. A representative from the Alliance of

Nurses for Healthy Environments talked about combining forces with a similarly motivated group from medicine, Physicians for Social Responsibility, which underscored Frost's point about the power of speaking across professions with a unified voice. Bringing these sorts of experiences into the classroom can show (rather than teach) that everyone has a story to tell and that whether it is at the federal, state, or local level, learners can see how "our voice counts," the participant said. Learning from other professions who were trained in how to do advocacy may also be a way of providing informal faculty development. With that thought, Carter moved to close the workshop, but not before Sheperis reminded the participants to think about their own commitments to learning and how, by developing an education contract with oneself, each health professional and educator can influence colleagues and leaners well after this workshop ends.

REFERENCES

NASEM (National Academies of Sciences, Engineering, and Medicine). 2019. *Integrating social care into the delivery of health care: Moving upstream to improve the nation's health*. Washington, DC: The National Academies Press.

Phillips, C. 2019. *Four years in the making, mental health center opens in south San Antonio school district*. Texas Public Radio. https://www.tpr.org/post/four-years-making-mental-health-center-opens-south-san-antonio-school-district (accessed January 23, 2020).

Appendix A

Members of the Global Forum on Innovation in Health Professional Education[1]

Caswell A. Evans, D.D.S., M.P.H. (*Co-Chair*)
National Academy of Medicine member
Associate Dean for Prevention and Public Health Services
University of Illinois at Chicago College of Dentistry

Deborah Powell, M.D. (*Co-Chair*)
National Academy of Medicine member
Professor, Department of Laboratory Medicine and Pathology
University of Minnesota

Frank J. Ascione, Pharm.D., M.P.H., Ph.D.
Director, University of Michigan Center for Interprofessional Education
Professor of Clinical and Social and Administrative Sciences
University of Michigan College of Pharmacy
Michigan Center for Interprofessional Education

David Benton, R.G.N., Ph.D., FFNF, FRCN, FAAN
Chief Executive Officer
National Council of State Boards of Nursing

---

[1] The National Academies of Sciences, Engineering, and Medicine's forums and roundtables do not issue, review, or approve individual documents. The responsibility for the published Proceedings of a Workshop rests with the workshop rapporteurs and the institution.

Reamer L. Bushardt, Pharm.D., PA-C, DFAAPA
Senior Associate Dean for Health Sciences
The George Washington University

Joanna M. Cain, M.D., FACOG
Professor and Vice Chair, Obstetrics and Gynecology
University of Massachusetts School of Medicine
American College of Obstetricians and Gynecologists

Robert Cain, D.O.
Chief Executive Officer
American Association of Colleges of Osteopathic Medicine

Kathy Chappell, Ph.D., R.N., FNAP, FAAN
Senior Vice President
Certification/Measurement, Accreditation, and Institute for Credentialing
    Research
American Nurses Credentialing Center

Steven Chesbro, PT, DPT, Ed.D.
Vice President for Education
American Physical Therapy Association

Amy Aparicio Clark, M.Ed.
Senior Program Officer, Cultivating Healthy Communities
Aetna Foundation

Darla Spence Coffey, M.S.W., Ph.D.
President
Council on Social Work Education

Darrin D'Agostino, D.O., M.P.H., M.B.A.
Executive Dean and Vice President of Health Affairs
Kansas City University
American Association of Colleges of Osteopathic Medicine

Jan de Maeseneer, M.D., Ph.D., FRCGP (Hon)
Chairman for European Forum for Primary Care Secretary-General
The Network: Towards Unity for Health
Vice-Dean for Strategic Planning at the Faculty of Medicine and Health
    Science
Ghent University (Belgium)

Marietjie de Villiers, Ph.D., M.B.Ch.B., M.Fam.Med., FCFP
Professor in Family Medicine
Deputy Dean, Education
Stellenbosch University

Kim Dunleavy, Ph.D., MOMT, P.T., OCS
Associate Clinical Professor
Director, Professional Education and Community Engagement
Department of Physical Therapy
University of Florida
American Council of Academic Physical Therapy

Kathrin (Katie) Eliot, Ph.D., R.D.
Director
Health Professions Educator
The University of Oklahoma Health Sciences Center
Academy of Nutrition and Dietetics

Sara E. Fletcher, Ph.D.
Vice President and Chief Learning Officer
Interim Chief Executive Officer
Physician Assistant Education Association

Jody Frost, P.T., D.P.T., Ph.D., FAPTA, FNAP
President-Elect
National Academies of Practice

Elizabeth (Liza) Goldblatt, Ph.D., M.P.A./H.A.
Director of Planning and Assessment
American College of Traditional Chinese Medicine
Board Chair
Academic Collaborative for Integrative Health

Catherine L. Grus, Ph.D.
Deputy Executive Director for Education
American Psychological Association

Anita Gupta, D.O., Pharm.D., M.P.P.
Senior Vice President, Medical Strategy and Government Affairs
Heron Therapeutics, Inc.

Kendra Harrington, PT, DPT, M.S.
Board-Certified Clinical Specialist in Women's Health Physical Therapy
Director, Residency/Fellowship Accreditation
American Board of Physical Therapy Residency and Fellowship Education
American Physical Therapy Association

Neil Harvison, Ph.D., OTR/L, FAOTA
Chief Academic and Scientific Affairs Officer
American Occupational Therapy Association

Eric Holmboe, M.D.
Senior Vice President
Milestones Development and Evaluation
Accreditation Council for Graduate Medical Education

Lisa Howley, M.Ed., Ph.D.
Senior Director of Strategic Initiatives and Partnerships
Association of American Medical Colleges

Holly Humphrey, M.D.
President
Josiah Macy Jr. Foundation

Emilia Iwu, M.S.N., R.N., APNC, FWACN
Ph.D. Scholar
Rutgers University

Pamela Jeffries, Ph.D., R.N., FAAN, ANEF
Dean of Nursing
The George Washington University

Phyllis M. King, Ph.D., OT, FAOTA, FASAHP
Associate Vice Chancellor for Academic Affairs University of
    Wisconsin–Milwaukee
Chair
Association of Schools of the Allied Health Professions

Sandeep "Sunny" Kishore, M.D., Ph.D., M.Sc.
President
Young Professionals Chronic Disease Network
Associate Director, Arnhold Institute for Global Health
Icahn School of Medicine at Mount Sinai

Kathleen Klink, M.D., FAAFP
Chief of Health Professions Education
Office of Academic Affiliations, Veterans Health Administration

Kathryn (Kathy) Kolasa, Ph.D., RDN, LDN
Professor Emeritus and Master Educator Department of Family
    Medicine–Nutrition and Patient Education
East Carolina University Brody School of Medicine
Academy of Nutrition and Dietetics

Kimberly Lomis, M.D.
Vice President for Undergraduate Medical Education Innovations
American Medical Association

Chao Ma, M.D.
Dean of Medical Education
Peking Union Medical College, Chinese Academy of Medical Sciences

Andrew Maccabe, D.V.M.
Executive Director
Association of American Veterinary Medical Colleges

Beverly Malone, Ph.D., R.N., FAAN
National Academy of Medicine member
Chief Executive Officer
National League for Nursing

Mary E. (Beth) Mancini, R.N., Ph.D., N.E.-B.C., FAHA, ANEF, FAAN
Associate Dean and Chair, Undergraduate Nursing Programs
Baylor Professor for Healthcare Research
The University of Texas at Arlington
College of Nursing
Past President
Society for Simulation in Healthcare

Dawn M. Mancuso, MAM, CAE, FASAE
Executive Director
Association of Schools and Colleges of Optometry

Angelo McClain, Ph.D., LICSW
Chief Executive Officer
National Association of Social Workers

Lemmietta G. McNeilly, Ph.D., CCC-SLP, CAE
Fellow
Chief Staff Officer, Speech-Language Pathology
American Speech-Language-Hearing Association

Mark Merrick, Ph.D., ATC, FNATA
Past President
Commission on Accreditation of Athletic Training Education
Athletic Training Strategic Alliance

Suzanne Miyamoto, Ph.D., R.N., FAAN
Chief Executive Officer
American Academy of Nursing

Warren Newton, M.D., M.P.H.
President and Chief Executive Officer Elect
American Board of Family Medicine

Loretta Nunez, M.A., Au.D., CCC-A/SLP, FNAP
Fellow
Director of Academic Affairs and Research Education
American Speech-Language-Hearing Association

David O'Bryon, J.D., CAE
President
Association of Chiropractic Colleges
Immediate-Past Chair
Academic Collaborative for Integrative Health

Bjorg Palsdottir, M.P.A.
Executive Director and Co-Founder
Training for Health Equity Network

Miguel Paniagua, M.D.
Medical Advisor, Test Materials Development
National Board of Medical Examiners

Rajata Rajatanavin, M.D., FAC
Minister of Public Health
Government of Thailand

Thomas Rebbecchi, M.D.
Medical Advisor, Marketing and Product Management
National Board of Medical Examiners

Jo Ann Regan, Ph.D., M.S.W.
Vice President of Education
Council on Social Work Education

Lucy A. Savitz, Ph.D., M.B.A.
Vice President, Research
Director, Center for Health Research, Oregon and Hawaii
Kaiser Permanente

Stephen Schoenbaum, M.D., M.P.H.
Special Advisor to the President
Josiah Macy Jr. Foundation

Joanne G. Schwartzberg, M.D.
Scholar-in-Residence
Accreditation Council for Graduate Medical Education

Wendi Schweiger, Ph.D., NCC, LPC
Director, International Capacity Building
Foundation and Professional Services
National Board for Certified Counselors, Inc. and Affiliates

Nelson Sewankambo, M.B.Ch.B., M.Sc., M.M.Ed., FRCP Doctor of Laws (HC)
National Academy of Medicine member
Principal and Professor
Makerere University College of Health Sciences

Javaid I. Sheikh, M.D., M.B.A.
Dean
Weill Cornell Medicine–Qatar

Carl J. Sheperis, Ph.D.
Dean, College of Education and Human Development
Texas A&M University–San Antonio

Susan E. Skochelak M.D., M.P.H.
National Academy of Medicine member
Vice President, Medical Education
American Medical Association

Jeffrey Stewart, D.D.S., M.S.
Senior Vice President for Interprofessional and Global Collaboration
American Dental Education Association

Zohray Talib, M.D.
Senior Associate Dean for Academic Engagement and Chair of Medical
    Education
California University of Science and Medicine

Maria Tassone, M.Sc.
Senior Director, Health Professions and Interprofessional Care, University
    Health Network
Director, Centre for Interprofessional Education, University of Toronto
*University of Toronto and University Health Network/Michener Institute
    of Education*

Melissa Trego, D.O., Ph.D.
Dean
Salus University, Pennsylvania College of Optometry
Association of Schools and Colleges of Optometry

Carole Tucker, Ph.D., M.S.
Associate Professor in the College of Public Health and the College of
    Engineering
Temple University
American Council of Academic Physical Therapy

Richard Weisbarth, O.D., FAAO, FNAP
Vice President, Professional Affairs for CIBA Vision Corporation
Alcon
President-Elect
National Academies of Practice

Karen P. West, D.M.D., M.P.H.
President and Chief Executive Officer
American Dental Education Association

Alison J. Whelan, M.D.
Chief Medical Education Officer
Association of American Medical Colleges

Adrienne White-Faines, M.P.A.
Chief Executive Officer
American Osteopathic Association

Launette Woolforde, Ed.D., DNP, R.N.-BC
Nursing Education and Professional Development Northwell Health
National League for Nursing

Xuejun Zeng, M.D., Ph.D., FACP
Chief and Associate Chair
Division of General Internal Medicine,
Peking Union Medical College Department of Medicine
Chinese Academy of Medical Sciences

Global Forum on Innovation in Health Professional Education Staff

Patricia Cuff, M.P.H., M.S.
Forum Director and Senior Program Officer
Board on Global Health

Katie Perez
Research Associate
Board on Global Health

Julie Pavlin, M.D., Ph.D., M.P.H.
Senior Director
Board on Global Health

*Forum sponsors and in-kind donors identified in italic.

Appendix B

Planning Meeting and Workshop Agendas

PLANNING MEETING AGENDA

Global Forum on Innovation in Health Professional Education Presents . . .
A discussion on the well-being of learners, trainees, faculty, and health professionals across the education-to-practice continuum and an information-gathering session on the social determinants of mental health: How do these two topics relate?

Come ready to share your thoughts on:
- How do we design systems that support the health and well-being of all health professionals and care providers?
- What is the role of leadership (administrative, education, health professional) in promoting and supporting action (not just words) to promote and support health and well-being?
- What are the social determinants of mental health?
- Are we supporting educators, learners, and care providers who work with victims of trauma? Are they themselves at risk of secondary trauma?

January 11, 2019

The National Academies of Sciences, Engineering, and Medicine's
Beckman Center
100 Academy Way, Irvine, CA 92617

7:30 a.m.   Registration and Continental Breakfast

8:00 a.m.   Welcome—Patricia Cuff, Director, Global Forum on
Innovation in Health Professional Education

**STRESS/BURNOUT AND WELL-BEING IN EDUCATION
AND PRACTICE**

8:10 a.m.   **Moderator:** Zohray Talib, California University of Science
and Medicine
Panel participants:
* Elizabeth Goldblatt, Academic Collaborative for
Integrative Health
* Ted Mashima, Association of American Veterinary
Medical Colleges
* Wendi Schweiger, National Board for Certified
Counselors

Open discussion to share

9:15 a.m.   **Break**

SOCIAL DETERMINANTS OF MENTAL HEALTH

9:30 a.m.   **Facilitator:** Zohray Talib, California University of Science
and Medicine

Describing the *social determinants of mental health*
* Carl Sheperis, National Board for Certified Counselors
  o Question for participants: How do you view the
    social determinants of mental health?

**Incorporating mental health into experiential education
about the social determinants**
* Share examples or ideas:
  o Stuart Gilman, Veterans Health Administration

  o Carol Mangione, University of California, Los Angeles (UCLA)–Care Harbor: The role of service learning in the educational process of health professionals

  o Kenneth Wells, UCLA, and Felica Jones, Healthy African American Families

  o Do **you** have an example or idea to share?

Supporting the well-being of students, faculty, and providers
- Wendi Schweiger, National Board for Certified Counselors
  - o Question for participants: How might the learner/faculty/provider be supported when working with those affected by the social determinants?

11:00 a.m. **Break**

11:15 a.m. **Review the planning committee's Statement of Task**
- Carl Sheperis, National Board for Certified Counselors

  Table discussion question 1: What are the urgent issues this workshop must address within the social determinants of mental health (consider the clinical learning environment)?

  Table discussion question 2: What suggestions might you give to the workshop planning committee that is tasked to build this workshop?

12:15 p.m. **ADJOURN TO LUNCH—All registered guests are invited**

WORKSHOP AGENDA

Educating Health Professionals to Address the Social Determinants of Mental Health: A Workshop

Global Forum on Innovation in Health Professional Education

November 14–15, 2019

**Keck Center of the National Academies, Room 100
500 Fifth Street, NW, Washington DC 20001**

WORKSHOP OBJECTIVE: To understand the physical and mental health impacts of being exposed to the social determinants from a macro and meso level so the knowledge can be applied in a micro level

DAY 1: NOVEMBER 14, 2019

Opening by Forum Co-Chair:
Caswell Evans, University of Illinois at Chicago

9:00 a.m.   **Welcome by workshop co-chairs**
- Kennita Carter, Health Resources and Services Administration, and Carl Sheperis, Texas A&M University

UNDERSTANDING THE SOCIAL DETERMINANTS—MACRO
Session Objective: To bring awareness to educators and practitioners that a person's mental and physical health are impacted by the social determinants and the two cannot be disentangled.

9:15 a.m.   **Social determinants of mental health across the lifespan**
- Ruth Shim, University of California, Davis

Q&A

10:00 a.m.   **A framework for educating health professionals to address the social determinants of health**
- Julian Fisher,* Hannover Medical School, Germany

10:10 a.m.   **Table exercise**
- Reflecting on living histories in terms of the social determinants of health
- Developing your own lifelong learning commitment to educating others about the social determinants of mental health

10:40 a.m.   **Break**

UNDERSTANDING THE SOCIAL DETERMINANTS OF
MENTAL HEALTH—MESO
Session Objective: To provide background and context
for exploring the development of an educational module
addressing the social determinants of mental health across
the life course.

11:00 a.m. Building a health workforce to address the social
determinants of mental health
Opening: Wendi Schweiger, National Board for Certified
Counselors
Moderator: Andrew Dailey, American Psychological
Association Minority Fellowship Program
- Panelist 1—Robert Horne, National Board for Certified
  Counselors Minority Fellow
- Panelist 2—Duy Nguyen, Council on Social Work
  Education Minority Fellowship Program
- Panelist 3—Dolores Subia BigFoot, American
  Psychological Association Minority Fellow

Facilitated discussion

12:30 p.m. **LUNCH**

1:30 p.m.   Educating the educator on an interprofessional approach
to addressing the social determinants of health through
education and action
Facilitators: Sandra Crewe, Howard University School of
Social Work, and Kathleen Klink, Office of Academic Affairs,
Veterans Health Administration
- Learning from the workshop participants

2:30 p.m.   **Break**

APPLYING MACRO AND MESO UNDERSTANDING
OF SOCIAL DETERMINANTS OF HEALTH/MENTAL
HEALTH TO MICRO APPROACHES

3:00 p.m.   Bringing education to life in and out of the classroom
Facilitator: Zohray Talib, California University of Science
and Medicine
Hearing from the community
Leader: Sandra D. Lane,* Syracuse University

Community members:
- Love Mouity, Catholic Charities
- Timothy "Noble" Jennnings-Bey, chief executive officer, Street Addictions Institute Inc.
  - o   What suggestions do you have for health professional educators who want to take their students out of the classroom to meet members of the community?

Hearing from health professions education students
Leader: Matthew Shank, President Emeritus, Marymount University
Students:
- Meghan Hamlin, School of Health Professions, Marymount University
- Molly Vencel, School of Nursing and Health Studies, Georgetown University
- Nigel Walker, Health Systems Management, George Mason University
  - o   What class had the greatest impact on you and why? And how might service-learning be made more effective from your perspective?

Hearing from health professions faculty providers
Leader: Warren Newton, American Board of Family Medicine
Faculty providers: Terri Lipman, University of Pennsylvania, School of Nursing
- o   How might you apply the points raised by students and community members to create transformative learning opportunities?

Panel discussion with the leaders
Moderator: Zohray Talib
- Community members leader: Sandra D. Lane
- Health professions education students leader: Matthew Shank
- Faculty providers: Warren Newton and Terri Lipman

4:30/   **Adjourn**
5:00 p.m.

DAY 2: NOVEMBER 15, 2019

Opening by Forum Co-Chair: Debra Powell, University of Minnesota

8:00 a.m. **Welcome by workshop co-chairs**
- Kennita Carter, Health Resources and Services Administration, and Carl Sheperis, Texas A&M University

Policy leaders driving mental health legislature and its impact on health professional education
- Moderator: David Benedek, Center for the Study of Traumatic Stress, Uniformed Services University of the Health Sciences
- Seth Moulton, U.S. House of Representatives, and former Marine officer

MICRO APPROACHES TO EDUCATING HEALTH PROFESSIONALS ON THE SOCIAL DETERMINANTS OF MENTAL HEALTH
Session Objective: Apply previous workshop discussions to exploring health professional education on the social determinants of mental health at three moments across the life course.

8:30/
8:45 a.m. **Breakout group instructions—Go to breakout room**
Discuss the social determinants of health education framework as it relates to mental health challenges described through living histories

8:45/
9:15 a.m. **Social determinants of mental health affecting perinatal mood disorders: Triggers of anxiety**
Gloria is a 27-year-old multipara female who presents to Rochester Regional Health in active labor with preterm premature rupture of membranes
- Leaders: Robert Keefe, University at Buffalo, and Emily Miller, Northwestern University

Social determinants of mental health challenges in young adulthood
Person X is between the ages of 18–21 years, in good physical health, presenting with suicidal ideations
- Leaders: Stephanie Townsell, American Osteopathic Association, and Mildred Joyner, President Elect, National Association of Social Workers

Social determinants of mental health issues touching older adults
Celia is a 78-year-old Boston woman who was admitted to the emergency room unable to walk after experiencing a work-related injury; she is otherwise in generally good health
- Leaders: Jorge Delva,* Boston University, and Melissa Batchelor-Murphy, Center for Aging, Health and Humanities, The George Washington University

10:00/ **Return to main room**
10:10 a.m.

10:15/ **Sparking thoughts and ideas**
10:30 a.m. • What activities can learners participate in, both in and out of the classroom, to learn about and affect the social determinants of mental health in the policy sphere?
- Revisiting your lifelong learning commitment to educating others about the social determinants of mental health

11:00 a.m. **Adjourn**

*Served on the National Academies committee that developed the framework for educating health professionals on the social determinants of health.

Appendix C

Speaker Biographical Sketches

Melissa Batchelor-Murphy, Ph.D., RN-BC, FNP-BC, FGSA, FAAN, is a tenured associate professor of nursing and a geriatric nursing researcher. She is the director of The George Washington University's interdisciplinary Center for Aging, Health and Humanities. Dr. Batchelor-Murphy has worked as an administrative nurse in skilled nursing homes and practiced as a family nurse practitioner (FNP) across long-term care settings. Her research, which is focused on patients with dementia, has been supported by The John A. Hartford Foundation, the Robert Wood Johnson Foundation Nurse Faculty Scholars program, and the National Institutes of Health/National Institute of Nursing Research. Dr. Batchelor-Murphy was previously an associate professor at Duke University and is board certified as a gerontological registered nurse and FNP. She is a fellow of the American Academy of Nursing and a 2017–2018 Health and Aging Policy Fellow serving the U.S. Senate Special Committee on Aging in the office of Senator Susan Collins.

Colonel David Benedek, M.D., received his B.A. from the University of Virginia in 1986 and his M.D. from the Uniformed Services University of the Health Sciences School of Medicine in 1991. After an internship and residency in psychiatry at the Walter Reed Army Medical Center, he was assigned as the division psychiatrist in the First Armor Division in Germany. From there, he deployed to the former Yugoslavia and delivered mental health support to U.S. and NATO Troops for Operation Joint Endeavor (1996). He returned to Walter Reed to complete forensic psychiatry fellowship training in 1998 and then served as the assistant chief of inpatient psychiatry. In 1999 he became the chief of Forensic Psychiatry Service and the director of the National Capital Consortium Military Forensic Psychiatry Fellowship Program at Walter Reed, and he remained in those positions until joining the Uniformed Services University of the Health Sciences Center for the Study of Traumatic Stress faculty in 2004. Dr. Benedek's awards include the Meritorious Service (2OLC) and Army Commendation (3OLC) Medals for his work at Walter Reed and in Bosnia, the LTG Claire Chennault Award for Outstanding Military Psychiatry Faculty Member, and the American Psychiatric Association's Nancy C.A. Roeske Award for Excellence in Medical Student Education. In 2002 he received the U.S. Army Surgeon General's "A" Proficiency Designator. He has authored or co-authored more than 75 scientific publications and has presented on numerous aspects of military, disaster, and forensic psychiatry at regional, national, and international professional conferences. He served on the American Psychiatric Association's (APA's) Committee on Confidentiality, was a consultant to APA's Practice Guideline for the treatment of acute stress disorder and posttraumatic stress disorder work-group in the development of its 2004 practice guideline, and the lead author of the 2009 guideline watch (update). He is the co-editor of the *Clinical Manual for Management of Posttraumatic Stress Disorder*. Dr. Benedek is a professor of psychiatry and the chairman of the Uniformed Services University of the Health Sciences' Department of Psychiatry, appointed in 2017. He is also an associate director of the University's Center for the Study of Traumatic Stress. He is a past president of the Society of Uniformed Service Psychiatrists, the Military District Branch of APA, and he is the currently the Society's deputy representative to the APA Assembly. He is a distinguished fellow of APA. In addition to his operational experience in Bosnia and Croatia, Dr. Benedek has deployed to Cuba, Iraq, and Kuwait in conjunction with the Global War on Terrorism. In 2004 he was appointed consultant to the U.S. Army Surgeon General for Forensic Psychiatry.

Dolores Subia BigFoot, Ph.D., a child psychologist, is a presidential professor who directs the Native American programs at the Center on Child Abuse and Neglect at The University of Oklahoma Health Sciences Center. Funded since 1994 by the Children's Bureau, she has directed the Project Making Medicine and, since 2003, the Indian Country Child Trauma Center, where she was instrumental in the cultural adaptations of evidence-based child treatments. Under her guidance, four evidence-based treatments were enhanced for American Indian and Alaska Native (AI/AN) families in Indian country, titled the Honoring Children Series. One of the four is Honoring Children—Mending the Circle, a cultural enhancement of trauma-focused cognitive behavioral therapy (TF-CBT) for use with AI/AN children and their families. Dr. BigFoot has more than 15 published articles and chapters, including serving as the lead author of *Adapting Evidence-Based*

Treatments for Use with American Indians and Native Alaskan Children and Youth. Dr. BigFoot has served as the principal investigator on 13 federally funded projects. Other distinctions include her service on the national advisory council of the Center for Mental Health Services at the Substance Abuse and Mental Health Services Administration, the National Network to Eliminate Health Disparities, and working groups for the Indian Health Service and the National Indian Child Welfare Association. She was selected to attend the White House conference on children's mental health and is the past president of the Society of Indian Psychologists. Dr. BigFoot has more than 30 years of experience and is knowledgeable about the concerns of implementation and adaptation of evidenced-based practices being introduced into Indian country. Dr. BigFoot is a member of the national TF-CBT Trainer Network. Dr. BigFoot is an enrolled member of the Caddo Nation of Oklahoma with affiliation to the Northern Cheyenne Tribe of Montana, where her children are enrolled members.

Kennita Carter, M.D., is a senior advisor in the Division of Medicine and Dentistry in the Bureau of Health Workforce at the Health Resources and Services Administration in the Department of Health and Human Services. She received a B.S. in psychobiology from the University of California, Los Angeles, and completed both medical school and a residency in internal medicine at the University of Maryland School of Medicine. She is a board-certified internist and fellowship-trained geriatrician. She completed her fellowship at the Union Memorial Hospital in Baltimore. She completed the Duke Integrative Leadership fellowship in Durham, North Carolina, and was a recipient of the Bravewell Leadership Fellowship in Integrative Medicine at the University of Arizona. She continues to serve as volunteer faculty training geriatric medicine fellows, internal medicine residents, and medical students in an interprofessional setting at the Department of Veterans Affairs. Other areas of interest include health equity, spirituality in medicine, and physician well-being.

Sandra Crewe, Ph.D., M.S.W., holds a B.S.W. and an M.S.W. from the National Catholic School of Social Services at The Catholic University of America. She earned her Ph.D. in social work from Howard University in Washington, DC. She is a member of the Academy of Certified Social Workers. Her research interests include family caregiving and kinship care (emphasis on older adults), program development and evaluation, and cultural competence. She has published articles in the *Journal of Human Behavior in the Social Environment, Affilia,* and the *Journal of Health and Social Policy*. She serves as the director of the Multidisciplinary Center for Social Gerontology. Dr. Crewe is a gubernatorial appointee for the Maryland Affordable Housing Trust; a member of the National Association of Housing and Redevelopment Officials (Resident Leadership Faculty); a member of the board of directors, American Association of Service Coordinators (chair professional development committee); an advisory council member of the Women's Health Institute and HIV/AIDS Consortium (Howard University); and a member and the chair of the ethnogeriatric and culture committee, Washington DC Area Geriatric Education Center Consortium (WAGECC). She is also a Master Faculty Scholar for WAGECC and a member of the National Association of Social Workers Aging Specialty Group and served as a member of the expert panel for Family Caregiving Standards. Dr. Crewe also serves on the Council of Social Work's professional development committee. She is a program evaluation/development consultant for the Department of Social Development (provincial government), Cape Town, South Africa.

Andrew Dailey, M.Div., M.S., has been with the Minority Fellowship Program (MFP) of the American Psychological Association since October 2002. He is responsible for the overall program, including the vision and mission of the MFP. Mr. Dailey works closely with federal funding agencies and advisory committees regarding policy decisions and serves as a liaison for the MFP's relationships with other organizations.

Jorge Delva, Ph.D., M.S.W., a nationally recognized expert on substance use disorders and ethnic health inequities, was appointed the dean of the School of Social Work at Boston University on January 1, 2018. Dr. Delva was the Kristine A. Siefert Collegiate Professor of Social Work and the director of the Communities Engagement Program of the Michigan Institute for Clinical and Health Research at the University of Michigan. He was a faculty associate in the Department of American Culture's Latina/o studies program. Dr. Delva conducts research focusing on addressing and reducing health inequities and helping improve the lives of low-income and racial and ethnic minority populations and communities. His areas of expertise include addictions and mental health, behavioral health, cross-cultural research, survey research, and community-based participatory research.

Julian Fisher, B.D.S., M.Sc., M.I.H., is a policy advisor and an analyst specializing in health workforce education, social and environmental determinants of health, and global oral health. He is currently based in Germany with regular trips to United Nations agencies in Switzerland. He is also the director of advocacy and network development in a part-time capacity for the nongovernmental organization Training for Health Equity, THEnet (New York). He holds a position as a research assistant professor in the Department of Public Health and Preventive Medicine at the SUNY Upstate Medical University in New York. As chair of two World Health

Organization (WHO) Technical Advisory Groups, he is engaged in supporting WHO's technical and normative work. Prior to this he was the associate director of professional and scientific affairs with FDI World Dental Federation in Geneva, Switzerland. His work experience covers a diverse range of professional domains, including international public health policy and advocacy (consultancies for WHO; the United Nations Educational, Scientific and Cultural Organization; and the United Nations Environment Programme), health profession (federation) management, and health workforce undergraduate and postgraduate education, both classroom and web based. His work has been based in geographical locations including Antarctica, Europe, Falkland Islands, Saudi Arabia, South Africa, and Tanzania within various sectors and organizations.

Robert A. Horne, Ph.D., serves as an assistant professor of counselor education and the director of the Addiction Studies Certificate Program at North Carolina Central University. Additionally, Dr. Horne serves as a counselor and a counseling consultant in private practice; a National Board for Certified Counselors mentor; and a fitness for practice evaluator for the North Carolina Board of Licensed Clinical Mental Health Counselors. Dr. Horne has previously served as the chair of the National Board for Certified Counselors Foundation Minority Fellowship Program Doctoral Advisory Council and as a subject-matter expert for the International Credentialing and Reciprocity Consortium. Dr. Horne holds a Ph.D. in counseling and counselor education from North Carolina State University, an M.A. in agency counseling from North Carolina Central University, and a master of divinity from Duke University. He is a National Certified Counselor, Licensed Clinical Mental Health Counselor, Approved Clinical Supervisor, Licensed Clinical Addiction Specialist, Certified Clinical Supervisor Intern, International Certified Advance Alcohol and Drug Counselor, and Master Addiction Counselor. Dr. Horne is a National Board for Certified Counselors fellow and a Substance Abuse Mental Health Service Administration fellow. Dr. Horne's research and publications focus on (1) African American male identity development and sustenance; (2) behavioral and substance addiction; and (3) spirituality, stress, coping, and cultural trauma. Dr. Horne actively engages in conducting national and international workshops, trainings, and webinars.

Timothy "Noble" Jennings-Bey resides in the city of Syracuse in upstate New York. Since 1996 Mr. Jennings-Bey has dedicated his life to working in the field of violence prevention. Currently, he is the director for the Trauma Response Team and the executive director of Street Addiction Institute Inc. (SAII Inc.). For more than a decade Mr. Jennings-Bey and his team have been on call 24 hours per day. The team responds to shootings and homicides while acting as a liaison among the Syracuse community, the Syracuse Police Department, and Upstate Medical Center. Mr. Jennings-Bey created SAII Inc. and the theory underlying it is that criminal activity specific to neighborhood violence has an addictive nature similar to alcohol, gambling, and substance abuse. Mr. Jennings-Bey believes that participants of gang and criminal activity are in need of respite and rehabilitation before they can be mainstreamed back into society. Syracuse University's Falk College has partnered with SAII Inc. to conduct research and offer families throughout the Syracuse community free counseling services specific to individuals affected by neighborhood violence. Mr. Jennings-Bey is a published author, mentor, consultant, and motivational speaker. His areas of expertise are trauma, grief and loss, depression, gang culture awareness, maladaptive behaviors, street addiction, and nontraditional intervention approaches specific to the street and gang culture.

Mildred Joyner, M.S.W., LCSW, BCD, has served as the director at DNB Financial Corporation since 2004. She has been the president of MCJ Consultants since January 2011 and is an emeritus professor of social work from West Chester University of Pennsylvania, where she started her teaching career in 1979. While at West Chester University she was elected in 1984 as the director and chairperson of the Undergraduate Social Work Program and served in that position until 2011. In 2010, Ms. Joyner chaired the fundraising committee for the Frederick Douglass sculpture that is permanently located on the campus of West Chester University. Ms. Joyner was elected in 2015 as the vice president of the National Association of Social Workers. She also serves on the boards of the Chester County Food Bank, the Dana-Farber Cancer Institute SoulMates advisory board in Boston, Massachusetts. She previously served on the boards of the Congressional Research Institute for Social Work and Policy in Washington, DC; the International Association of Schools of Social Work; the ANSWER Coalition; Chester County Children, Youth, and Families; the Chester County Women's Commission; and the Council on Social Work Education (CSWE) in Alexandria, Virginia, and as the president and the board chair from July 2010 to June 2013. Ms. Joyner is a chair emeritus of Living Beyond Breast Cancer in Narberth, Pennsylvania, where she previously served as the board chair and as the chair of Board Governance. In addition, Ms. Joyner also served as the vice president of CSWE, and is a past president of the Association of Baccalaureate Social Work Program Directors, a national organization located in Alexandria, Virginia. Ms. Joyner earned her B.S.W. in 1971 from Central State University in Ohio and an M.S.W. in 1974 from Howard University in Washington, DC.

Robert Keefe, Ph.D., MSSA, joined the University at Buffalo School of Social Work faculty as an associate professor in 2005 from Syracuse

University. Passionate about public health social work, community health, and health and disability, Dr. Keefe possesses several years of post-M.S.W. health and mental health care practice experience as a medical and psychiatric social worker in facilities in New Hampshire and Ohio and as a case manager/clinical care reviewer in New York. He is also a member of the American Public Health Association, Society for Social Work and Research, National Association of Social Workers, and Council on Social Work Education. In addition to teaching several courses centering on mental health, health, and interventions, Dr. Keefe is also the faculty liaison and academic advisor for the M.S.W./M.P.H. dual degree program. With his current project, "Postpartum Depression Among New Mothers of Color," funded by the Fahs-Beck Foundation of the New York Community Trust, Dr. Keefe endeavors to help service providers render culturally competent services to new mothers of color. His significant contributions to the field have earned him high honors; in addition to being selected as the Public Health Social Worker of the Year by the American Public Health Association in 2011, he was also named a fellow of The New York Academy of Medicine in 2013. Dr. Keefe received his Ph.D. from the University at Albany's School of Social Welfare subsequent to earning an MSSA from Case Western Reserve University and a B.A. in sociology from Ithaca College.

Kathleen Klink, M.D., FAAFP, is the chief of health professions education in the Office of Academic Affiliations in the Department of Veterans Affairs. She is responsible for overseeing all of the clinical trainee portfolios of the Veterans Health Administration, including advanced fellowships, associated health education, medical and dental education, and nursing education. She has served as the director of the Center for Family and Community Medicine at the Columbia University College of Physicians and Surgeons, the chief of Service for Family Medicine at NewYork–Presbyterian Hospital, a Robert Wood Johnson Health policy fellow in the Office of Senator Hillary Rodham Clinton, the director of the Division of Medicine and Dentistry in the Bureau of Health Professions at the Health Resources and Services Administration, and the medical director of the Robert Graham Center for Policy Studies in Family Medicine and Primary Care. Dr. Klink most recently served as the director of medical and dental education in the Office of Academic Affiliations. Dr. Klink is a board-certified family physician. A graduate of the University of Miami School of Medicine, she completed her residency at the Jackson Memorial Hospital/University of Miami. She has devoted most of her career caring for underserved people and advocating for improved access through enhanced workforce training that provides vulnerable populations services where and when the need is greatest.

Sandra D. Lane, Ph.D., M.P.H., is the Laura J. and L. Douglas Meredith Professor of Teaching Excellence and a professor of public health and anthropology at Syracuse University, and a research professor in the Department of Obstetrics and Gynecology at Upstate Medical University. She received her Ph.D. in medical anthropology from the joint program at the University of California, San Francisco, and Berkeley, and an M.P.H. in epidemiology from the University of California, Berkeley. Her research focuses on the impact of racial, ethnic, and gender disadvantage on maternal, child, and family health in urban areas of the United States and the Middle East. Dr. Lane has published 52 peer-reviewed journal articles; 23 book chapters; a 2008 book titled *Why Are Our Babies Dying? Pregnancy, Birth and Death in America*; and a policy monograph, *The Public Health Impact of Needle Exchange Programs in the United States and Abroad*. Her work has been funded with 10 federal grants (from the National Institute of Mental Health, the Centers for Disease Control and Prevention, the Environmental Protection Agency, the Health Resources and Services Administration, and the Office of Minority Health) in addition to foundation and state grants and several internal grants. In addition to the Meredith award, she received the Carl F. Wittke Award for Distinguished Undergraduate Teaching and the John S. Diekhoff Award for Distinguished Graduate Teaching, both at Case Western Reserve University. Dr. Lane has developed a model that links the community-participatory analysis of public policy with pedagogy, called CARE (Community Action Research and Education). Her CARE projects include food deserts in Syracuse, lead poisoning in rental property, health of the uninsured, and her current project on neighborhood trauma and gun violence. Her CARE publications since joining the Syracuse University faculty have included as co-authors 22 community members and 75 students (not an unduplicated list because some students and community members were participants more than once). Prior to joining Syracuse University, Dr. Lane was the founding director of Syracuse Healthy Start, an infant mortality prevention program, in Syracuse, New York. She was a Ford Foundation program officer for child survival and reproductive health in the Middle East and has also been a consultant to the World Health Organization for operational research on tuberculosis, the United Nations Population Fund and the United Nations Children's Fund for Rapid Assessment Procedures, and the Joint Commission on the Accreditation of Healthcare Organizations for qualitative methods in hospital evaluation. Dr. Lane was also the 2015 recipient of the Henrik L. Blum Award for Excellence in Health Policy from the American Public Health Association and the 2020 George Foster Award for Practicing Medical Anthropology from the Society for Medical Anthropology.

Terri Lipman, Ph.D., CRNP, MSN, is the assistant dean for community engagement, the Miriam Stirl Endowed Term Professor of Nutrition and

Professor of Nursing of Children at the University of Pennsylvania School of Nursing, a senior fellow in the Center for Public Health Initiatives, and a distinguished fellow of the Netter Center for Community Partnerships. Her research is currently focused on disparities in the care and outcomes of children with diabetes—with an emphasis on addressing the social determinants of health—and on gender disparities in the evaluation of linear growth. She was funded by the National Institute of Child Health and Human Development at the National Institutes of Health to study an academic–community partnership to increase activity in youth and their families and by the Children's Hospital of Philadelphia to integrate community health workers into care of underserved children with chronic disorders.

Emily Stinnett Miller, M.D., M.P.H., is professionally trained as an obstetrician and a maternal–fetal medicine physician. She has formal training in study design and epidemiologic analysis through the completion of a master's in public health. Her research focuses on obstetric and perinatal outcomes related to perinatal mental health disorders, and she has dedicated her career to optimizing the treatment of perinatal depression. Her unwavering commitment to improving perinatal mental health care is evidenced by her involvement in several projects that have advanced health care delivery in the area of perinatal depression. Collaborating with mental health experts, she has contributed to a chapter on mental health in one of the preeminent obstetric textbooks. She was nominated to the American College of Obstetricians and Gynecologist's Maternal Mental Health Expert Workgroup to develop a consensus statement to guide care provision for perinatal depression and anxiety and obstetrician-facing decision support. In recognizing gaps in health care services, she challenged the paradigm of the current obstetric model of perinatal depression care and received a Friends of Prentice Special Projects Initiative Award to implement a collaborative care model for perinatal depression support services (COMPASS) at Northwestern University. In the 2.5 years since COMPASS launched, more than 1,300 women have been referred for mental health collaborative care. Adherent to the core principles of collaborative care, COMPASS has made a positive impact in the lives of hundreds of pregnant and parenting women. The footprint of COMPASS has expanded beyond individual patient care; COMPASS has changed the culture of obstetric care at Northwestern, empowering obstetricians and midwives to take ownership of depression screening and treatment by the development of educational resources and clinical tools for depression care. COMPASS is now expanding beyond the walls of Northwestern, providing guidance on successful collaborative care implementation strategies to other academic sites across the United States.

Love H. Mouity is a former refugee from the Republic of the Congo who has had great experiences working in different companies since coming to the United States. He was able to gain useful experience and now works at Catholic Charities of Onondaga at the Refugee Resettlement Program as one of the health services program coordinators. He participated in Mental Health First Aid USA courtesy of the National Council for Behavioral Health in January 2019. He is an alum of the Community College of Onondaga and Syracuse University at the Maxwell School of Citizenship and Public Affairs. He co-teaches the refugee health course, which is a collaborative project of Upstate Medical University, Syracuse University, and Catholic Charities of Syracuse.

Seth Moulton was first called to service when he joined the Marines in 2001, days after graduating from college and months before the attacks on 9/11. As the leader of an infantry platoon, he was among the first Americans to reach Baghdad in 2003. He served four tours in a war that he did not agree with—but he was proud to go, so that no one had to go in his place. After returning home from Iraq, Mr. Moulton earned joint degrees in business and public policy at graduate school and then worked in the private sector in Texas to build the country's first high-speed rail line. But it was not long before he was called to serve once again—this time in his home district in Massachusetts. Mr. Moulton ran—and won—on a platform of bringing a new generation of leadership to Washington, DC, becoming the only Democrat to unseat an incumbent in a primary in 2014. In the two terms since he was first sworn in, Representative Moulton has worked tirelessly to uphold his commitment to bipartisanship. He has passed several bipartisan bills, including the Faster Care for Veterans Act and the Modernizing Government Travel Act, and he was named the most effective freshman Democrat by the Center for Effective Lawmaking. He has also concentrated on spurring economic development in Massachusetts, creating the first intergovernmental task force focused on growing the economy of Lynn, the biggest city in his district. Today, as a member of the House Committee on the Budget, Representative Moulton is focused on creating a new economic agenda that will make a difference for American families. He also sits on the House Committee on Armed Services and is the top Democrat on the House Subcommittee on Oversight and Investigations.

Warren Newton, M.D., M.P.H., serves as the president and the chief executive officer (CEO) for the American Board of Family Medicine (ABFM). As president and CEO of ABFM, he also oversees the ABFM Foundation and the Pisacano Leadership Foundation. Dr. Newton previously served as the executive director of the North Carolina Area Health Education Center (NC AHEC), a national leader in practice redesign, continuing professional development, health careers programming, and innovation in graduate medical education, and he was the vice dean of education at the University of North Carolina (UNC) School of Medicine. From 1999 to 2016 he served as the William B. Aycock Professor and Chair of Family Medicine at UNC. Dr. Newton has served as a personal physician for 34 years, working in a variety of settings, including the UNC Family Medicine Center, the Moncure Community Health Center, and the Randolph County Health Department. In the 1990s he founded the first hospitalist program at UNC Hospitals and helped reorganize family medicine obstetrics into a maternal child service. For the past 15 years he led practice transformation initiatives at the practice, regional, and statewide levels; NC AHEC now provides ongoing support for health information technology, patient-centered medical home, and quality improvement for more than 1,200 primary care practices. Dr. Newton graduated from Yale University in 1980 and Northwestern Medical School in 1984. After residency and chief residency at UNC, he completed the Robert Wood Johnson Foundation Clinical Scholars Program and an M.P.H. at UNC. In 2012–2013 he served as a Society of Teachers of Family Medicine Bishop fellow, during which he also completed the American Council of Education fellows program.

Duy Nguyen, Ph.D., LCSW, M.S.W., is the director of the Substance Abuse and Mental Health Services Administration–funded Minority Fellowship Program at the Council on Social Work Education. A gerontological mental health services researcher, his grant-funded research has revealed how sociocultural factors, especially differences among Asian ethnic groups and the aging process, affect health and mental health service use. As an educator, he has held faculty appointments at Columbia University, New York University, and Temple University, where he has taught courses in research, statistics, and human behavior in the social environment. A licensed clinical social worker, Dr. Nguyen earned his B.A. and M.S.W. from Washington University in St. Louis and his Ph.D. from Columbia University. He is a fellow of the Gerontological Society of America and the Society for Social Work and Research.

Wendi K. Schweiger, Ph.D., NCC, LPC, is the director of international capacity building at the National Board for Certified Counselors, Inc. & Affiliates (NBCC). In this position, Dr. Schweiger organizes and facilitates NBCC's collaboration efforts with counselors and counseling organizations outside the United States that are taking steps to professionalize. She has worked for NBCC in a variety of capacities and was named to her current position in September 2018. Dr. Schweiger has been a National Certified Counselor since 1998. She is a Licensed Professional Counselor in North Carolina and an inductee of the Chi Sigma Iota honor society. She travels, presents, and trains worldwide, and she has co-authored publications inside and outside of the United States. Dr. Schweiger completed her undergraduate studies at Salem College in Winston-Salem, North Carolina. She earned her Master of Science and Educational Specialist degrees in community counseling in 1997 and her doctorate in counselor education in 2008 at the University of North Carolina at Greensboro.

Matthew Shank, Ph.D., became the eighth president of the Virginia Foundation of Independent Colleges (VFIC) in January 2019. The mission of VFIC is to advance the distinctive values and strengths of 15 independent member colleges and universities in Virginia. Prior to his tenure at VFIC, Dr. Shank served as the interim president of the World Affairs Council in the District of Columbia. Previously, Dr. Shank became Marymount University's sixth president in July 2011 and stepped down to become president emeritus in June 2018 after 7 years of service. In recognition of his work at Marymount, Dr. Shank received the 2012 Global Education Leadership Award from the World Affairs Council. In addition, he accepted the World Affairs Council–DC Global Educator of the Year Award on behalf of Marymount in March 2017. He has also received the Robert Ball Lifetime Achievement Award from the Ballston Business Improvement District in 2018 and the Edu-Futuro Community Partner Award in 2017 and earned the distinction of visiting distinguished professor at the National University of Public Service in Budapest, Hungary, in 2016. Dr. Shank currently serves on a variety of nonprofit boards, including Arlington Free Clinic (advisory); Arlington Public Schools (advisory); Arlington Street Peoples Assistance Network; American University in the Emirates, Dubai; Cristo Rey High School in Washington, DC; Dream Project (advisory); Leadership Center for Excellence (advisory); National Catholic Education Association; Northern Virginia Community College Foundation; 4Stay; and Women's Foundation of Washington, DC. An accomplished scholar, Dr. Shank has published numerous articles, presented at many conferences, and is the author of *Sports Marketing: A Strategic Perspective* (5th edition). He has consulted with more than 75 organizations in the areas of marketing research, strategic planning, and marketing strategy.

Carl Sheperis, Ph.D., M.S., is the dean at Texas A&M University–San Antonio. Previously Dr. Sheperis was the interim president and the chief executive officer of the National Board for Certified Counselors, Inc. and Affiliates (NBCC) and its division NBCC International. Headquartered in Greensboro, North Carolina, NBCC is the preeminent certification agency for professional counselors in the United States. It has certified more than 64,000 counselors and provides licensure examinations for all 50 states, the District of Columbia, Puerto Rico, and Guam. Dr. Sheperis completed his undergraduate studies at Kutztown University in Pennsylvania. He earned a Master of Science in Education in 1994 from Duquesne University and his doctorate in mental health counseling in 2001 from the University of Florida. He is a national certified counselor, certified clinical mental health counselor, master addictions counselor, approved clinical supervisor, and licensed professional counselor, as well as a past NBCC board chair. Before joining NBCC full time in April 2018, he was the program dean for the College of Social Sciences at the University of Phoenix, and earlier served at Lamar University in Beaumont, Texas, where he was the chair of the Counseling and Special Populations Department and led the largest state university system counseling program in the United States. Dr. Sheperis has been the president of the Association for Assessment and Research in Counseling and an associate editor for the *Journal of Counseling and Development*, as well as serving as the editor of the *Journal of Counseling Research and Practice*. He has also worked with the American Counseling Association as the chair of the Research & Knowledge Committee.

Ruth Shim, M.D., M.P.H., holds the Luke & Grace Kim Professorship in Cultural Psychiatry in the Department of Psychiatry and Behavioral Sciences at the University of California (UC), Davis, School of Medicine. She is an associate professor of clinical psychiatry, the director of cultural psychiatry, and the chair of the Vice Chancellor's Advisory Committee on Faculty Excellence in Diversity at UC Davis Health. She is a member of the board of trustees of the Robert Wood Johnson Foundation and a co-editor of *The Social Determinants of Mental Health*.

Zohray Talib, M.D., FACP, is the senior associate dean for academic affairs and the chair of medical education at the California University of Science and Medicine. Dr. Talib is a member of the National Academies of Sciences, Engineering, and Medicine's Global Forum on Innovation in Health Professional Education and also holds academic appointments at the Aga Khan University in Kenya as well as the Mbarara University of Science and Technology in Uganda. Dr. Talib's research focuses on strategies to strengthen medical and health professions education in low-resource settings and for underserved communities. She was the medical education lead and co-investigator for the Coordinating Center of the Medical Education Partnership Initiative, working with medical schools in Africa, examining training models aimed at improving the quantity, quality, and retention of graduates. She has published on medical education innovations and strategies to support the scale-up of training programs for underserved communities. Dr. Talib is also an advocate for gender parity in global health leadership and has written commentaries that bring light to this issue in both *The Lancet* and *The Lancet Global Health*. Dr. Talib has led global health initiatives in Central Asia and East Africa ranging from community-based cancer screening to research training for academic faculty. She brings to the field of global health the unique perspective of being a primary care clinician, educator, and researcher. She was previously an associate professor of medicine and health policy at The George Washington University, where she held leadership positions in undergraduate and graduate medical education. Dr. Talib received her B.S. in physical therapy from McGill University in Montreal, Canada, and her M.D. from the University of Alberta in Edmonton, Canada. She completed her residency in internal medicine at The George Washington University Hospital. She is board certified by the American Board of Internal Medicine and a fellow of the American College of Physicians.

Stephanie Townsell, M.P.H., serves as the director of public health for the Department of Research & Development at the American Osteopathic Association. In this role, she is directly responsible for the development and implementation of public health initiatives and policies as well as other research and educational initiatives of the organization. Prior to this role, Ms. Townsell was the director of HIV surveillance for the Chicago Department of Public Health, where she managed multiple Centers for Disease Control and Prevention grants aimed at monitoring the HIV epidemic, analyzing collected data, and disseminating findings to community and clinical stakeholders. Additional public health experiences include facilitation of faith-based prevention and awareness programs, management of evaluation research projects, and coordination of the Community Engagement and Research Core of the Center for Clinical and Translational Sciences at the University of Illinois. She is also an active member of the Community Engagement Advisory Board for the University of Illinois and an ambassador and a grant reviewer for the Patient-Centered Outcomes Research Institute. Ms. Townsell is personally and professionally very passionate about social justice issues impacting vulnerable populations. She has specific interest in addressing health inequity, the elimination of health disparities, and advocating for the overall health and well-being of families and individuals in high-poverty communities. For many years, she and her family have lived on the Westside of Chicago, in one of the poorest neighborhoods in the country. They proudly joined with others to relocate and engage in efforts to rebuild the community and redistribute financial resources to address the need. Ms. Townsell and her family are partners in a coalition aimed at creating affordable housing, quality health care, after-school programs, and transitional housing to formerly incarcerated persons, and organizing neighbors to address pressing social problems. Her neighbors' issues are not theoretical. Every day she sees neighbors who are self-medicating with alcohol and other substances; people who are hurting, frustrated, and hopeless. She learned from her own experience growing up the value of having people present in one's life to encourage and challenge your vision for the future, listen, and provide support. So she and her family made a goal to help provide the same for others. Ms. Townsell holds a B.S. in chemical engineering from Northwestern University and an M.P.H. from the University of Illinois at Chicago School of Public Health in maternal and child health/epidemiology.

Appendix D

Background Paper

SOCIAL DETERMINANTS OF MENTAL HEALTH

According to the World Health Organization (WHO) and Calouste Gulbenkian Foundation, the social determinants of mental health (SDMH) involve the economic, social, and political conditions into which one is born that dictate the likelihood a person raised in poverty will develop persistent mental health challenges throughout his or her life (WHO and Calouste Gulbenkian Foundation, 2014). While the term is somewhat new, the concept of linking poverty to mental health disorders dates back at least to 2003, when Patel and Kleinman linked mental disorders with education and poor housing (Patel and Kleinman, 2003). Despite knowing the associations, and despite the recent focus many health professional schools are placing on educating students about the physical health effects of the social determinants, addressing the underlying causes of mental health disorders remains a gap in the education of most health professionals outside of the mental health and social service professions. Given the growing divide between rich and poor, as cited by the Organisation for Economic Co-operation and Development (OECD, 2015), the existence of well-trained health professionals who can advocate for their patients with mental health challenges is becoming increasingly essential.

EDUCATION

A review of the literature uncovered articles describing the SDMH, but none of them offered guidance to faculty on how to incorporate key issues into their curriculum (Allen et al., 2014; Ssebunnya et al., 2009; WHO and Calouste Gulbenkian Foundation, 2014). The National Academies of Sciences, Engineering, and Medicine (NASEM, 2016) published a framework for educating health professional students to address the social determinants. Similarly, Doran and colleagues (2008) detailed their curriculum on social determinants—known as the Poverty in Healthcare Curriculum—which was designed for medical students at the University of Michigan. While neither set of authors mentioned the mental health aspects of the social determinants, they did lay out a structure that could guide educators on how to set up a social determinants curriculum. Both examples drew inspiration from Kolb's experiential learning theory as described by Rooks and Rael (2013). Such education would use experiential learning opportunities combined with observation and reflection to encourage learners to become actively involved in the SDMH. While that describes how educators could guide learners, a more pressing question is how—if at all—educators are currently educating students on the SDMH. For those who report educating their students on aspects of poverty and mental health, the next question is whether any evaluation of their classes or assessments of their learners was conducted to determine the impact of their education on individuals and/or communities.

PRACTICE

Poverty is a key driver of those social determinants that are strongly associated with experiencing traumatic life events (Luby et al., 2013). These events range across the lifespan from unsupportive parenting and inadequate nutrition to being victims of physical and psychological abuse. Such events can have permanent detrimental impacts on the victims. Bak and Hvidhjelm (2017) explained trauma-informed care as an approach to setting up mental and physical safety nets for survivors who have experienced trauma. Similarly, trauma-informed practice supports providers who have experienced secondary trauma. Emergency medical teams and social and mental health workers recognize the importance of preventing and managing primary and secondary trauma across the education-to-practice continuum. Other health professions appear to acknowledge that secondary trauma is an issue but do not purposefully educate their students, faculty, or health professionals on how to address their own mental health challenges. In addition, many care organizations are not equipped with appropriate services and policies that would encourage healing for those exposed to trauma.

REFERENCES

Allen, J., R. Balfour, R. Bell, and M. Marmot. 2014. Social determinants of mental health. *International Review of Psychiatry* 26(4):392–407.

Bak, J., and J. Hvidhjelm. 2017. The pros and cons of implementing trauma informed care in Danish psychiatry. *Violence in Clinical Psychiatry,* edited by P. Callaghan, N. Oud, H. Nijman, T. Palmstierna, and J. Duxbury. Amsterdam, The Netherlands: Oud Consultancy. Pp. 125–129.

Doran, K. M., K. Kirley, A. R. Barnosky, J. C. Williams, and J. E. Cheng. 2008. Developing a novel Poverty in Healthcare curriculum for medical students at the University of Michigan Medical School. *Academic Medicine* 83(1):5–13.

Luby, J., A. Belden, K. Botteron, N. Marrus, M. P. Harms, C. Babb, T. Nishino, and D. Barch. 2013. The effects of poverty on childhood brain development: The mediating effect of caregiving and stressful life events. *JAMA Pediatrics* 167(12):1135–1142.

NASEM (National Academies of Sciences, Engineering, and Medicine). 2016. *A framework for educating health professionals to address the social determinants of health.* Washington, DC: The National Academies Press.

OECD (Organisation for Economic Co-operation and Development). 2015. *Income inequality: The gap between rich and poor.* OECD Insights. https://doi.org/10.1787/9789264246010-en (accessed January 28, 2020).

Patel, V., and A. Kleinman. 2003. Poverty and common mental disorders in developing countries. *Bulletin of the World Health Organization* 81(8):609–615.

Rooks, R. N., and C. T. Rael. 2013. Enhancing curriculum through service learning in the social determinants of health course. *Journal of the Scholarship of Teaching and Learning* 13(2):84–100.

Ssebunnya, J., F. Kigozi, C. Lund, D, Kizza, and E, Okello. 2009. Stakeholder perceptions of mental health stigma and poverty in Uganda. *BMC International Health and Human Rights* 31(9):5.

WHO (World Health Organization) and Calouste Gulbenkian Foundation. 2014. *Social determinants of mental health.* World Health Organization. https://apps.who.int/iris/bitstream/handle/10665/112828/9789241506809_eng.pdf;jsessionid=0038B0C30674BF3E2FB51AA66F11B74F?sequence=1 (accessed January 28, 2020).

Appendix E

Faculty Development Materials

EDUCATING FACULTY ON THE MENTAL HEALTH IMPACTS OF THE SOCIAL DETERMINANTS

1

Educating Faculty on the Mental Health Impacts of the Social Determinants

Social Determinants of Mental Health

2

Definition

The social determinants of mental health (SDMH), involve the economic, social and political conditions into which one is born that dictate the likelihood a person raised in deficient or dangerous conditions often associated with poverty will develop persistent mental health challenges throughout his or her life (WHO and Calouste Gulbenkian Foundation, 2014).

Adapted from the World Health Organization (WHO) and the Calouste Gulbenkian Foundation (2014).

3

Learning Objectives

After this workshop, participants will be able to:

1. Understand the impact of the social determinants of mental health across the lifespan
2. Understand how mental health can be incorporated into the HPE framework for the social determinants of health
3. Differentiate the impact of the social determinants on physical and mental health at macro, meso, and micro levels
4. Examine opportunities to expand health professional education to incorporate the social determinants of mental health
5. Identify experiential learning opportunities related to the social determinants of mental health for health professional education
6. Design a framework for delivering education on the social determinants of mental health to health professionals-in-training
7. Implement strategies for health professional education that incorporate the social determinants of mental health

4

SDMH Highlights

- It is not just the physical health *or* the mental health of a person that requires support; moving forward, health professionals must bring together the mind and body so learners and practitioners can recognize the importance of caring for the whole person. (Sheperis)
- The social determinants of mental health deserve equal attention to the social determinants of physical health because mental health conditions have high costs, prevalence, morbidity, and mortality, and they have been neglected in conversations about social determinants. (Shim)
- All policies have an impact on people's mental and physical health, and health professionals have a responsibility to advocate for policies that will improve health. (Shim)
- There is a lack of mental health incorporation into health professional education outside of the mental and behavioral health professions. (Sheperis & Talib)

What are the social determinants of health (SDH)?   5

SDH is defined as "those factors that impact upon health and wellbeing: the circumstances into which we are born, grow up, live, work, and age, including the health system" (CSDH, 2008).

- The SDH, said Shim, are predominantly responsible for the health disparities and health inequities that are seen both within and between countries. These terms – disparities and inequities – are often confused, although they are distinct concepts:
- **Health disparities:** differences in health status among distinct segments of the population including differences that occur by gender, race or ethnicity, education or income, disability, or living in various geographic localities.
- **Health inequities:** disparities in health that are a result of systemic, avoidable, and unjust social and economic policies and practices that create barriers to opportunity.

The impact of social determinants   10

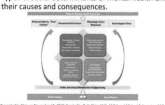

The difference between equality and equity   6

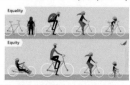

SOURCE: Presented by Shim on November 14, 2019; RWJF. 2017. Visualizing health equity: One size does not fit all infographic. https://www.rwjf.org/en/library/infographics/visualizing-health-equity.html (accessed January 22, 2020). Copyright 2017. Robert Wood Johnson Foundation. Used with permission from the Robert Wood Johnson Foundation.

Types of social determinants of mental health and their causes and consequences.   11

SOURCE: Presented by Shim on November 14, 2019; Created by Ruth Shim, M.D., M.P.H. and Michael T. Compton, M.D., M.P.H.

SDH Outcomes   7

Derived from a children's game of "why"?

- Why is Jason in the hospital? - Because he has a bad infection in his leg.
- But why does he have an infection? - He has a cut on his leg and it got infected.
- But why does he have a cut on his leg? He was playing in a junk yard next to his apartment building and fell on some sharp, jagged steel there.
- But why was he playing in a junk yard? His neighborhood is run down. Kids play there and there is no one to supervise them.
- But why does he live in that neighborhood? His parents can't afford a nicer place to live.
- But why can't his parents afford a nicer place to live? His dad is unemployed and his mom is sick.
- But why is his dad unemployed? Because he doesn't have much education and he can't find a job.
- But why....?

Source: Government of Canada. 2013. What makes Canadians healthy or unhealthy? https://www.canada.ca/en/public-health/services/health-promotion/population-health/what-determines-health/what-makes-canadians-healthy-unhealthy.html (accessed January 22, 2020)

From Knowledge to Action: Highlights   12

- Contained in National Academies' report on *Educating health professionals to address the social determinants of mental health* was the need to emphasize experiential learning that is interprofessional and cross-sectoral. (Fisher)
- Both learners and practitioners need to practice in such a way that acknowledges and addresses the social determinants of mental health, or the health professions will never get beyond where they are now. (Klink)
- One of the challenges [to using a team-based model of care] was trying to change the dynamics of a team of health professionals who are used to working parallel to each other in silos...policy issues will have to be addressed if a sustainable interprofessional environment that bridges academia and practice is to be created. (Carter)
- As educators seek to bring SDMH into the classroom, it is important that they examine their own biases, conscious and unconscious, in order to better guide their students toward addressing disparities that can increase joy in their patients' lives. (Crewe)

Poor mental health outcomes   8

Poor mental health outcomes, said Shim, have been associated with multiple social determinants, including adverse childhood experiences, discrimination, poverty, unemployment, income inequality, food insecurity, and the built environment.

Framework for lifelong learning   13

SOURCE: NASEM (National Academies of Sciences, Engineering, and Medicine). 2016. A framework for educating health professionals to address the social determinants of health. The National Academies Press. doi: 10.17226/21923

Separating MH disorders from SDH   9

Mental health (MH) disorders are particularly difficult to separate from social determinants, said Shim, because conditions are "filtered through the lens of society" and diagnoses are, in large part, based on observations and interpretations of behavior.

Behaviors may have different underlying reasons, but these reasons are often not considered when making a diagnosis.

For example, said Shim, a child who is hyperactive and disruptive in class may be diagnosed with attention deficit hyperactivity disorder. However, these behaviors may be more readily explained by the fact that the child is hungry. Social determinants such as food insecurity may not only be associated with mental health disorders, but may in fact be confounded with them.

Small group activity   14

Divide into small groups to further discuss innovative models with an emphasis on the challenges of implementing interprofessional education focused on the social determinants and mental impacts.

Recruiting and Supporting a Diverse Workforce: Highlights   15

- A diverse health workforce, drawn from the community that it serves, is best suited to help the community and patients address social determinants of mental health. (Horne)
- The Minority Fellowship Program (MFP) was created in 1973 in order to increase the number of ethnic minorities in mental health professions and to provide more culturally competent care to an increasingly ethnically diverse population in the United States. (Schweiger)
- The MFP builds on this [shared experience] by affirming and validating the fellows' life experiences, building a space where fellows can be authentic, promoting self-efficacy, building community, and empowering creativity. (Nguyen)
- The main role of a mentor is forging a path that supports the mentee in achieving as much as possible. (BigFoot)

Critical elements   16

. . . for recruiting, supporting, retaining, and promoting a diverse workforce include:

- Organizational support
- Opportunity to be authentic
- Support for students and professionals
- Integration with community
- Mentorship
- Community definitions of well-being and success
- Self-care and support

Experiential learning in and out of the Classroom: Highlights[17]

- Experiential learning requires a community that is ready and receptive to building partnerships; students who are engaged and motivated to make a difference, and faculty who are committed to doing the hard work to bring communities and students together. (Talib)
- It can be difficult for refugees to open up about their past, so people working with them must take the time to gain trust in order to build a relationship of mutual honesty and openness. (Mouity)
- When building relationships between academia and communities, it is critical that faculty members be intentional and sincere...Communities can sense if an academic is "trying to meet a quota" or check the boxes for community engagement. (Jennings-Bey)
- [The students] all agreed that community- and project-based classes were preferable to traditional classes... [but] that not all students are passionate about the same things, so schools should offer varying levels of engagement and the ability to choose projects that meet students' interests. (Walker, Hamlin, Vencel)
- An academic could team up with a practitioner in order to run a community-based project giving students the opportunity to learn different aspects of the work from different people. (Shank)
- Community-based learning opportunities need to be flexible, based on community needs and goals, and need to be part of a long-term commitment between communities, institutions, faculty, and students (Lipman)

Community perspective   18

- In the classroom: Love Mouity moved to Syracuse, New York as a refugee from Congo-Brazzaville in 2007. He now works as a coordinator for refugee outreach for Catholic Charities of Onondaga County, and also co-teaches an interprofessional class at Syracuse University on refugee health.
- Out of the classroom: Timothy "Noble" Jennings-Bey is CEO of the Street Addictions Institute Inc. and Director for the Trauma Response Team, which responds to shootings and homicides in Syracuse, New York. Jennings-Bey grew up in Syracuse in a low-income, violent neighborhood, and now serves as a leader in his community and works closely with academics and students at Syracuse University.

Interprofessional collaborations   19

- Student perspective: Walker said that his program has been largely theory and classroom-based, so learning with students who participate in more real-life experiences (e.g. working in a clinic) would bring a much-needed balance to the program.
- University president perspective: Shank added that another option for interprofessional education is to have instructors from different disciplines working together with traditional health professions faculty. For example, an academic could team up with a practitioner in order to run a community-based project, giving students the opportunity to learn different aspects of the work from different people.

Turning Experience into Policy: Highlights   20

- Many Veterans chose not to use the word "disorder" [in the post-traumatic stress acronym] citing that after what they went through in battle, it would be a disorder not to be affected by the experience. (Moulton)
- It was also stated that, in the end, legislation and public policy may help the most—even more than the delivery of quality health care—in reducing these inequities. (Benedek)
- Putting the patient in the center means seeing the whole person—including his or her family, job, community, and unique situation—rather than just his or her medical issue or diagnosis. (Keefe)
- Health professionals need to be prepared and willing to work cross-sectorally in order to address social determinants. (Carter)
- Students need to be trained to see "health in all policies" and to advocate for all types of policy on all levels, (Fisher)

Role of health education in policy   21

- Leverage the skillsets of other professions like counseling, social work, and psychology, for interprofessional education and training in policy advocacy
- Offer a broad continuum of engagement in advocacy, with a core foundation of advocacy skills that all students are trained in.
- Examples:
  - take students to a state capitol or to Capitol Hill for advocacy days & train students in how to:
    - write letters to influence policy;
    - know who their representatives are; and
    - use their "voice" in terms of policy development.

Closing   22

Think about your own commitments to learning and how, by developing an education contract with yourself, how you as a health professional and/or an educator can influence colleagues and leaners well after this workshop ends.

CASE HISTORY 1

Social Determinants of Mental Health Affecting Perinatal Mood Disorders: Triggers of Anxiety

---

1

Social Determinants of Mental Health Affecting Perinatal Mood Disorders: Triggers of Anxiety

Case History of Gloria[1]

Presented by
Robert Keefe, University at Buffalo
Emily Stinnett Miller, Northwestern University

[1]NOTE: This case history has been fictionalized for educational purposes

---

5

Given the medical history, are you comfortable with discharging Gloria?

2

Activity Agenda

10 minutes - Opening & introductions
20 minutes - Discuss case study
20 minutes - Small group activity
10 minutes - Large group discussion

6

Social History – Rounding Update

- Gloria lived and worked in inner city Rochester, NY her entire life
- Her grandparents moved to this neighborhood from NYC in 1961
- Her parents had an 8th grade education
- She and her 5 siblings all dropped out of high school
- Married for 8 years
- Just prior to the birth, Gloria was in a motor vehicle accident

---

3

Medical History – Rounding Update

- Gloria is a 27 year old G3P2 who presented to Rochester Regional Health in labor at 36 weeks 1 day gestation
  - History of diabetes and hypertension
  - Reports active use of marijuana and tobacco
- Progressed quickly in labor and had a vaginal delivery
- At delivery a large retro-placental clot was noted
  - EBL = 800mL
- Several clinicians noted Gloria did not seem to appear to understand discussions pertaining to prematurity or her excessive blood loss

---

7

Do you have any questions for Gloria before you discharge her?

4

SDMH Highlights

- It is not just the physical health or the mental health of a person that requires support; moving forward, health professionals must bring together the mind and body so learners and practitioners can recognize the importance of caring for the whole person. (Sheperis)
- The social determinants of mental health deserve equal attention to the social determinants of physical health because mental health conditions have high costs, prevalence, morbidity, and mortality, and they have been neglected in conversations about social determinants. (Shim)
- All policies have an impact on people's mental and physical health, and health professionals have a responsibility to advocate for policies that will improve health. (Shim)
- There is a lack of mental health incorporation into health professional education outside of the mental and behavioral health professions. (Sheperis & Talib)

8

Social History – Rounding Update

- Relationships
  - Reginald is Gloria's husband; Hx of incarceration; No steady employment/low-paying jobs; Has 3 children not with Gloria
  - No friend or family support
  - Cares for 2 children and now 1 newborn
  - Feels supported by her health center
- Living situation
  - High-crime neighborhood
  - Recently evicted

The motor vehicle accident

"[O]ne day we were driving to Walmart. And she seen us in the car together...with our kids. And she ...jumped out her car window... [W]e tried to lock all the doors, but he didn't get the last back door. And she got in, and she punched me in the stomach probably like eight times. Telling me 'I'm gonna kill the baby'. That scared the hell out of me. ...that day, all my fluids leaked.... they rushed me into the hospital, and then I had [my daughter] ...that same day."

List the social determinants that affected Gloria 12

1. Living in poverty
2. History of domestic violence
3. Living in a high-crime neighborhood
4. Living in inner-city, dilapidated housing
   1. Lead-based paint
   2. History of bug infestations
   3. Passive toxic exposures from car fumes
5. 10th grade education
6. Few friends or supports
7. Family of origin is dysfunctional

10

What were the social determinants that affected Gloria?

Small Group Activity   13

- Form 3 teams by counting 1,2,3
  - Team 1 goes to the first easel
  - Team 2 goes to the second easel
  - Team 3 goes to the third easel
- Record your responses on the flip chart – add to the other groups' responses
- Each group gets [5min] to discuss the question and record their responses before moving to the next easel

---

List the social determinants that affected Gloria 11

1. _____
2. _____
3. _____
4. _____

Reconvene in Large Group   14

1. How did social determinants affect Gloria's physical and mental health?

2. What are the intergenerational affects of the social determinants on Gloria and her newborn/older children?

3. What activities can students do in and out of the classroom to learn about and affect the social determinants of mental health during pregnancy in the policy sphere?

CASE HISTORY 2

Social Determinants of Mental Health Challenges in Young Adulthood

1

Social Determinants of Mental Health Challenges in Young Adulthood

Case History of Person X[1]

Presented by:
Stephanie Townsell, Director of Public Health, American Osteopathic Association
Mildred "Mit" Joyner, President-elect, National Association of Social Workers

[1]NOTE: This case history has been fictionalized for educational purposes

---

Activity Agenda   **2**

5 minutes   Introductions
5 minutes   Opening remarks
5 minutes   Present Person X case
15 minutes   Activity
20 minutes   Activity discussion
10 minutes   Reflect upon health professional
             education & policy

Key Concepts   **3**

Health	A state of complete physical, mental, and social well-being, not simply the absence of sickness and disease (WHO, 2014).
Social determinants of health	"Conditions in the environments in which people are born, live, learn, work, play, worship, and age that affect a wide range of health, functioning, and quality-of-life outcomes and risks" (Healthy People, 2019). • Includes factors such as socioeconomic status, education, neighborhood and physical environment, employment, and social support networks, as well as access to health care. • Shaped by the distribution of money, power, and resources (WHO, 2014). • Mostly responsible for health inequities (Healthy People, 2019).
Structural determinants	Root determinants, such as historical, political, ideological, economical, and social foundations, from which all other determinants arise (WHO, 2010).

Case: Person X   **4**

• Between the ages of 18-21 years.
• Presents with suicide ideations.
• Originally referred for a mental health assessment.

History   **5**

• Father was admitted to the hospital with Peritonitis for the fourth time in two months.
• Referring discharge planner needed to determine if Person X could adequately provide care for father.
• Dad was in end stages of kidney disease; required dialysis three times a week.

History   **6**

• Family was advised to a skilled nursing home placement unless someone in family could care for father full time.
• Entire family emphatically rejected nursing home placement.
• Person X finally agreed to take on the full responsibility and medical care needs for the father.
• When supportive services were offered to the family, the family declined.

History   **7**

What we know:
• Person X is the oldest member in a family of five.
• Person X recently came out to the family (only). The family refuses to talk about Person X's sexual preference.
• Person X is enrolled in a prestigious university pre-med program, received numerous academic honors and awards, as well as a full academic scholarship.
• Person X is first generational and has a strong affiliation with the Que's and recently decided to join.

History   **8**

• Person X has missed several classes and academic success is spiraling downward over the last few weeks.
• No one in the program knows that Person X is now taking care of the father full time, and Person X feels compelled to help the mother and siblings.
• Person X refuses to talk to anyone about the family's current circumstances. In fact, the entire family is engaged in numerous family secrets.

History 9

- Person X does not live at home.
- Mother and father recently separated; the father moved out.
- Siblings live with the mother and have not been very supportive or assisted with day-to-day medical needs of the Dad.

14

Compare and Contrast Figures

History 10

- Mother currently holds membership in Jack and Jill.
- Both parents are active members of the Links.
- Father is a member of the Boule and is a Knight.

Discussion 15

- What could be inferred about Person X based on the history?
- Name the social determinants affecting Person X?
- How did they impact Person X?

History 11

- Person X recently revealed to the mental health clinician that all Person X can think about every day is planning the father's home-going services.
- Person X feels it may be easier on everyone if Person X and the Dad were no longer around.

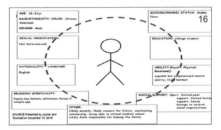

Activity 12

- Give Person X a name.
- Write what you know about Person X on the stick figure provided.
- Include social determinants of mental health related to Person X and Person X's family.
- What community supports does Person X already have? What supports might you recommend?

Key Concept 17

| Intersectionality | Overlap and interdependence of various social identities, such as race, gender, sexuality, and class, contributes to the specific type of systemic oppression and discrimination experienced by an individual |

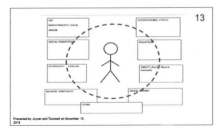

Discussion 18

- What assumptions did you make about Person X?
- Why were those assumptions made?
- Were any assumptions erroneous?
- Could they alter how Person X is engaged, cared for, or treated?

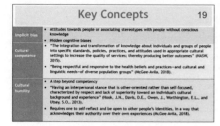

	Key Concepts 19
Implicit bias	• Attitudes towards people or associating stereotypes with people without conscious knowledge • Hidden cognitive biases
Cultural competence	• "The integration and transformation of knowledge about individuals and groups of people into specific standards, policies, practices, and attitudes used in appropriate cultural settings to increase the quality of services; thereby producing better outcomes" (NASW, 2015). • "Being respectful and responsive to the health beliefs and practices—and cultural and linguistic needs of diverse population groups" (McGee-Avila, 2018).
Cultural humility	• A step beyond competency • "Having an interpersonal stance that is other-oriented rather than self-focused, characterized by respect and lack of superiority toward an individual's cultural background and experience" (Hook, J.N., Davis, D.E., Owen, J., Worthington, E.L., and Utsey, S.O., 2013). • Requires one to self-reflect and be open to other people's identities. In a way that acknowledges their authority over their own experiences (McGee-Avila, 2018).

Discussion   20

- What biases can you identify?
- How might they impact Person X?

Discussion   21

- What activities can learners participate in, both in and out of the classroom, to learn about and affect the social determinants of mental health among young adults in the policy sphere?

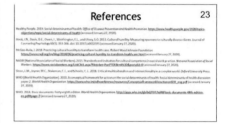

Questions?
Comments?

References   23

Healthy People. 2019. Social determinants of health. *Office of Disease Prevention and Health Promotion.* https://www.healthypeople.gov/2020/topics-objectives/topic/social-determinants-of-health (accessed January 27, 2020).

Hook, J.N., Davis, D.E., Owen, J., Worthington, E.L., and Utsey, S.O. 2013. Cultural humility: Measuring openness to culturally diverse clients. *Journal of Counseling Psychology* 60(3): 353-366. doi: 10.1037/a0032595 (accessed January 27, 2020).

McGee-Avila, J. 2018. Practicing cultural humility to transform health care. *Robert Wood Johnson Foundation.* https://www.rwjf.org/en/blog/2018/06/practicing_cultural_humility_to_transform_health_care.html (accessed January 27, 2020).

NASW (National Association of Social Workers). 2015. Standards and indicators for cultural competence in social work practice. *National Association of Social Workers.* https://www.socialworkers.org/LinkClick.aspx?fileticket=PonPTDEBrmY%3D&portalid=0 (accessed January 27, 2020).

Sloan, L.M., Joyner, M.C., Stakeman, C.J., and Schmitz, C.L. 2018. Critical multiculturalism and intersectionality in a complex world. *Oxford University Press.*

WHO (World Health Organization). 2010. A conceptual framework for action on the social determinants of health: Social determinants of health discussion paper 2. *World Health Organization.* https://www.who.int/sdhconference/resources/ConceptualframeworkforactiononSDH_eng.pdf (accessed January 27, 2020).

WHO. 2014. Basic documents: Forty-eighth edition. *World Health Organization.* http://apps.who.int/gb/bd/PDF/bd48/basic-documents-48th-edition-en.pdf?ua=1 (accessed January 27, 2020).

CASE HISTORY 3

Social Determinants of Mental Health Issues Touching Older Adults

---

1

Social Determinants of Mental Health
Issues Touching Older Adults

Case History of Cecilia[1]

Presented by
Jorge Delva, School of Social Work and Center for Innovation in
Social Work & Health, Boston University

Melissa Batchelor-Murphy, Center for Aging, Health and Humanities,
GW School of Nursing

[1]NOTE: This case history has been fictionalized for educational purposes

---

5

Now that she's medically
stable, is there any reason
not to discharge her?

2

Activity Agenda

10 minutes - Opening & introductions
20 minutes - Discuss case study
20 minutes - Small group activity
10 minutes - Large group discussion

6

Do you have any
questions for Cecilia
before you discharge her?

3

Social History - Rounding Update

Cecilia is a 77 year old woman who has worked her
entire life. She recently stopped working due to a
work-related injury. She lives alone.

- Cecilia has lived in her home city all her life
- She rents a 1-bedroom apartment in her home city
- Rent has gone up in her neighborhood

7

Social History - Rounding Update

- **Relationships**
  - Cecilia's husband died 10 years ago
  - She has no family support - her 2 siblings passed away; she has a niece
    that she is not in touch with; her only child died young of cancer
  - She is not connected with any churches
- **Living situation**
  - Rising rent in her neighborhood
  - Recently evicted

4

Medical History - Rounding Update

Cecilia is a 78 year old woman
who was admitted with an acute
metatarsal fracture of her right
foot after a computer was
dropped on it. She also has
arthritis that she mostly controls
with nonsteroidal anti-
inflammatory drugs, and mildly
high blood pressure that she
usually takes diuretics for.

Cecilia's blood pressure and pain
are now under control. She is
medically stable and ready for
discharge. The social worker will
work with her on discharge
planning, with instructions to get
a walker and a follow-up
appointment with orthopedics in
[2] weeks

8

Social History - Rounding Update
Meet Cecilia

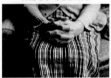

SOURCE: Photo from Pixabay; reprinted under Pixabay License.

9

What were the
social determinants
that affected Cecilia?

Reconvene in Large Group   12

1. How might the social determinants have affected Cecilia's physical and mental health?

2. In what ways do the social determinants affect the elderly differently than at other points along the life course?

3. What activities can students do in and out of the classroom to learn about and to address the social determinants of mental health of elderly populations in the policy sphere?

List the social determinants that affected Cecilia   10

1. _____

2. _____

3. _____

4. _____

For more information and   13
additional faculty
development materials,
please contact
ihpe@nas.edu

The National Academies of
SCIENCES · ENGINEERING · MEDICINE

Small Group Activity   11

- Form 3 teams by counting 1,2,3
  - Team 1 goes to the first easel
  - Team 2 goes to the second easel
  - Team 3 goes to the third easel
- Record your responses on the flip chart – add to the other groups' responses
- Each group gets [5min] to discuss the question and record their responses before moving to the next easel

Appendix F

Forum-Sponsored Products

**GLOBAL FORUM ON INNOVATION IN HEALTH PROFESSIONAL
EDUCATION SUMMARIES AND PROCEEDINGS**

nationalacademies.org/ihpeglobalforum

*Interprofessional Education for Collaboration: Learning How to Improve
Health from Interprofessional Models Across the Continuum of Education
to Practice: Workshop Summary* (2013)

Establishing Transdisciplinary Professionalism for Improving Health Outcomes: Workshop Summary (2013)

Assessing Health Professional Education: Workshop Summary (2013)

*Building Health Workforce Capacity Through Community-Based Health
Professional Education: Workshop Summary* (2014)

*Empowering Women and Strengthening Health Systems and Services
Through Investing in Nursing and Midwifery Enterprise: Lessons from
Lower-Income Countries: Workshop Summary* (2015)

*Measuring the Impact of Interprofessional Education on Collaborative
Practice and Patient Outcomes* (2015)

Envisioning the Future of Health Professional Education: Workshop Summary (2015)

A Framework for Educating Health Professionals to Address the Social Determinants of Health (2016)

Exploring the Role of Accreditation in Enhancing Quality and Innovation in Health Professions Education: Proceedings of a Workshop (2016)

Future Financial Economics of Health Professional Education: Proceedings of a Workshop (2017)

Exploring a Business Case for High-Value Continuing Professional Development: Proceedings of a Workshop (2018)

Improving Health Professional Education and Practice Through Technology: Proceedings of a Workshop (2018)

A Design Thinking, Systems Approach to Well-Being Within Education and Practice: Proceedings of a Workshop (2019)

Strengthening the Connection Between Health Professions Education and Practice: Proceedings of a Joint Workshop (2019)

The Role of Nonpharmacological Approaches to Pain Management: Proceedings of a Workshop (2019)

NATIONAL ACADEMY OF MEDICINE PERSPECTIVE PAPERS

Breaking the Culture of Silence on Physician Suicide (2016)

I Felt Alone But I Wasn't: Depression Is Rampant Among Doctors in Training (2016)

Defining Community-Engaged Health Professional Education: A Step Toward Building the Evidence (2017)

100 Days of Rain: A Reflection on the Limits of Physician Resilience (2017)

A Multifaceted Systems Approach to Addressing Stress Within Health Professions Education and Beyond (2017)

Addressing Burnout, Depression, and Suicidal Ideation in the Osteopathic Profession: An Approach That Spans the Physician Life Cycle (2017)

Burnout, Stress, and Compassion Fatigue in Occupational Therapy Practice and Education: A Call for Mindful, Self-Care Protocols (2017)

Promoting Well-Being in Psychology Graduate Students at the Individual and Systems Levels (2017)

Stress-Induced Eating Behaviors of Health Professionals: A Registered Dietitian Nutritionist Perspective (2017)

Breaking Silence, Breaking Stigma (2017)

Breaking the Culture of Silence: The Role of State Medical Boards (2017)

The Role of Accreditation in Achieving the Quadruple Aim (2017)

Nursing, Trauma, and Reflective Writing (2018)

The Role of Health Care Profession Accreditors in Promoting Health and Well-Being Across the Learning Continuum (2018)

Utilizing a Systems and Design Thinking Approach for Improving Well-Being Within Health Professions' Education and Health Care (2019)

Compassionate, Patient-Centered Care in the Digital Age (2019)